# PREVENTION OF HEALTH PROBLEMS

**Dr.J.M. Shah. Ph.D (Alt. Med.).**

www.jmshah.com

STARDOM BOOKS

WORLDWIDE

www.StardomBooks.com

**STARDOM BOOKS**

A Division of Stardom Publishing

and infoYOGIS Technologies.

105-501 Silverside Road

Wilmington, DE 19809

First edition July 2015


Prevention of health problems,
by DR.J.M. SHAH. Ph.D (Alt. Med.)

p. cm.


1. Health & Fitness / Alternative Therapies I. Title


ISBN-13: 978-1515353553
ISBN-10: 1515353559

# DEDICATION

Dedicated to my wife Surekha for inspiration in my research work.

# DISCLAIMER

# Note from the Publisher

It was a great pleasure to work with all the CO-AUTHORS of this book to bring out their stories, perspectives and insights on how they did what they did.

Each one of them have gone through their own struggles, overcome challenges and successfully steered their businesses and careers into becoming a well-known names in their respective industries.

Through this publication, I wanted to bring out their views so that you, the reader can benefit and get inspired by their achievements. The experts were specifically asked to share how they did what they did and their message to the world.

So, here it is, for not just your reading pleasure, but also as a reference guide to help you shorten the learning curve and outshine in your own personal endeavors.

As you are going to learn by reading from the contributors of this book, you will understand that all of them have one common thing to say… TAKE ACTION.

Go ahead, read the book, take action and bring about a positive difference in your life, business and career – today!

WHEN YOU ARE RIGHT AND OTHERS ARE WRONG...
-- BE FORGIVING AND CONSIDERATE
WHEN YOU ARE WRONG AND OTHERS ARE RIGHT...
-- BE APOLOGETIC AND COURAGEOUS
..BECAUSE IT TAKES A LOT OF COURAGE TO BE SORRY AND
APOLOGIZE.

## RAAM ANAND, PUBLISHER

# CONTENTS

# 1

## HOW TO REMAIN

## HEALTHY, HAPPY AND PROSPEROUS

### - BY JASHVANT SHAH, CHAIRMAN & MANAGING DIRECTOR OF SURU GROUP OF COMPANIES.

Being a Pharmacy Graduate, I was interested in preventing health problems instead of treating diseases, as it is said that prevention is better than cure.

I consulted many medical practitioners, but could not get any medicine for prevention of major Health Problems of Heart, Lungs, Liver, Kidney or Brain.

I therefore took support of alternative medicine.

Four systems of Alternative Medicine

**1. Aura and Aura Photography**

**2. Gems Therapy**

**3. Dowsing**

**4. Prayers**

1. Aura and Aura Photography

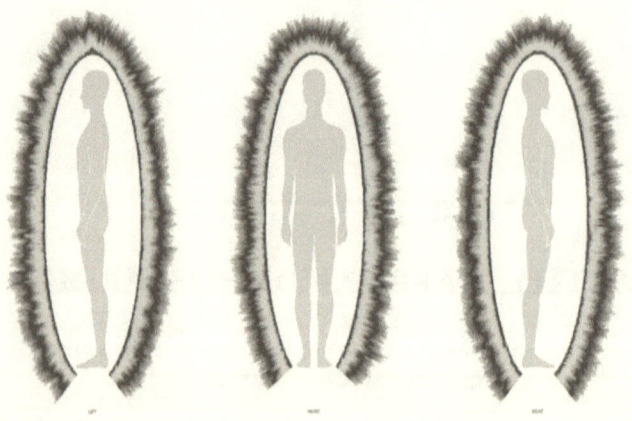

All living beings have auric body. It is a Vibrational body surrounding our physical body. Dark energy at above times enter our auric body and brings us unhappiness and invite disease.

Aura is a light force of the soul. When soul enters body at the time of birth, body starts vibrating and starts its functions. At the time of death soul leaves the body Aura vanishes and vibrations subside.

All living forces including plants, insects, creature are having soul, without soul there is no vibrations and no Aura. Seven layers of the Auric body system represent seven layers of atmospheres of our plant earth. As these atmospheric layers of the earth protect it from the outside evasions of foreign bodies, same way seven layers of Auric body protect the living being from negative or dark energies and diseases.

## The Myth and Science of Kirlian Photography

Kirlian photography, although the study of which can be traced back to the late 1700s, was officially invented in 1939 by Semyon Davidovitch Kirlian. The Kirlian photographic process reveals visible "auras" around the objects photographed. These photographs have been the subject of much controversies over the years. Interestingly, much of this was initially put forth by the inventor himself, along with his wife to explain the Kirlian photography phenomena.

Kirlian photography is also known as Aura Photography. To understand Aura Photography one should know what is aura. We have two bodies: one is physical visible body and another invisible auric body. For example people doing meditation have a glow on their face. This is aura.

The aura or energy field reflects the powerful connection our brain and nervous system create between the body, mind and spirit. A person's thoughts, emotions and beliefs are mirrored in the aura, which is why the aura and chakras can be used to determine underlying issues related to physical symptoms. In the year 2000, another Russian scientist Dr. Konstantin Korotkov updated this camera to directly record, process and interpret aura images with a computer. This camera is known as GDV Camera.

### Therapeutic Use

The most common therapeutic use of Kirlian photography is as a diagnostic tool. Variations in the shapes, colours and intensity of images produced are said to provide clues to the patients overall health and energy level. It indicates presence or absence of diseases, specific emotional states and other physiological or psychological conditions.

### Scientific Research

Results of scientific experiments published in 1976 involving Kirlian photography of living tissue (human finger tips) showed that most of the variations in corona discharge streamer length, density, curvature and color can be accounted for by the moisture content on the surface of and within the living tissue.

Konstantin Korotkov developed a technique similar to Kirlian photography called Gas Discharge Visualization (GDV). Korotkov's GDV camera system consists of hardware and software to directly record, process and interpret GDV images with a computer.

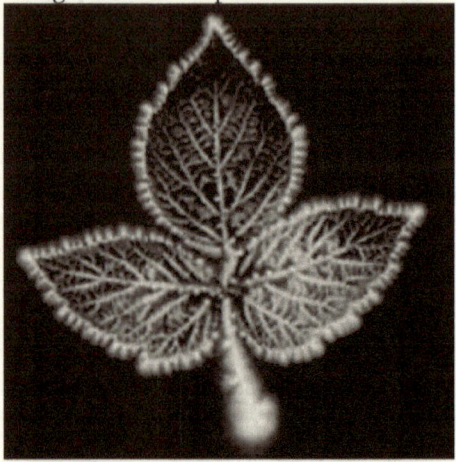

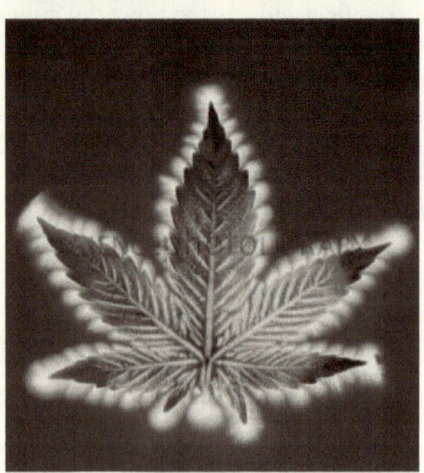

## How Kirlian Photography Helps Healers

Many common eastern medicine traditions including Reiki and acupuncture are based on energy fields in the body. Kirlian photography, because it gives a practioner the ability to visualize these energy fields is a useful diagnostic and evaluative tool.

Acupuncturists can, for example take aura photography of a person during an initial evaluation and see especially where the energy is out of balance. It is not a replacement for acupuncturist's traditional diagnostics skills but rather a supplement and a way for them to demonstrate their assessment to a patient visually.

Scientists and practioners also theorize that Kirlian photography has a role in detecting cancer and other devastating diseases. For example, plants with cancer shows up with a very vivid carona or electrical field than healthy plants. This is due to the high metabolic rate of cancerous cells.

Kirlian Photography may also be able to treat patients under psychiatric care. The images has the ability to exhibit the emotional state of the person being photographed.

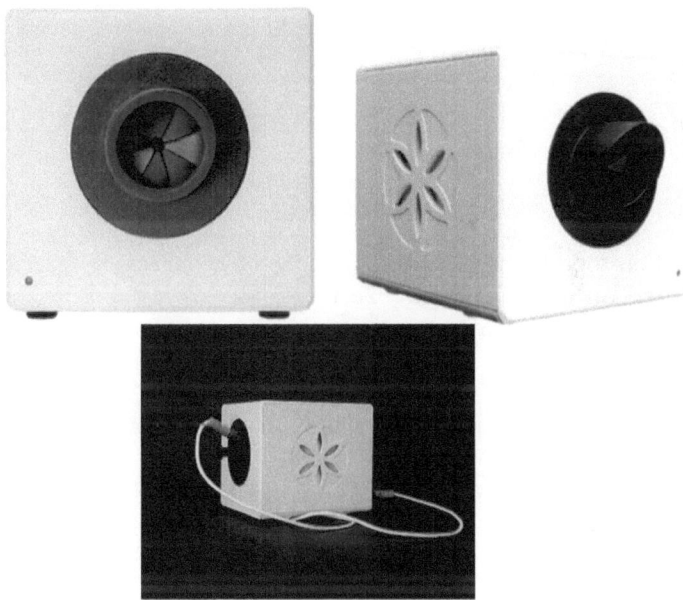

### An Example

Given below is the Aura Photograph of Sachin Bhilare who is suffering from Asthma and indigestion and is prone to heart problems.

The right side diagram shows problem with respiratory system & problem with duodenum indicated by peaks of blue line & red line.

Left side diagram shows problem with right part of heart, coronary vessels, respiratory system & transverse colon.

Energy Status

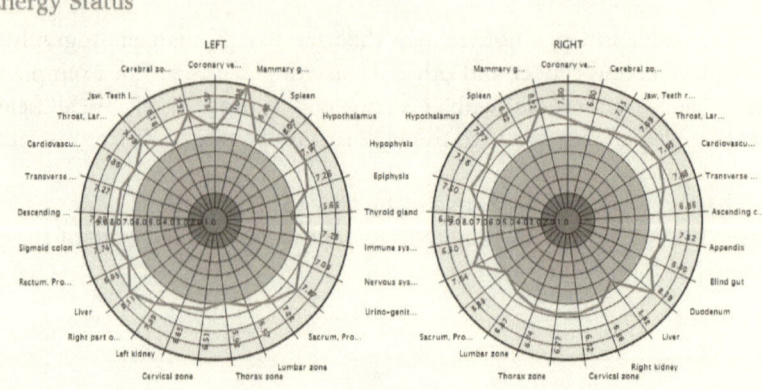

## Procedure

The process of taking a Kirlian photo is a fairly simple one and does not even require the use of a camera. First, a sheet of photographic film is placed on top of a metal plate. Then, the object that is to be photographed is placed on top of the film. To create the initial exposure, high voltage current is applied to the metal plate. The electrical coronal discharge between the object and the metal plate is captured on the film. The Kirlian photograph, which shows a light, glowing silhouette around the photographed object, becomes visible as a result of developing the film.

Although the Kirlians invented this photographic process in 1939, they didn't publicly release information about their experiments until 1958, and Kirlian photography wasn't a well-known phenomenon to the general public until 1970.

In GDV Camera, we have to place fingers of both right hand left hand on camera lens. Auric energy of these fingers are registered in the computer and software develops aura photograph of the person.

## 2. Gems Therapy

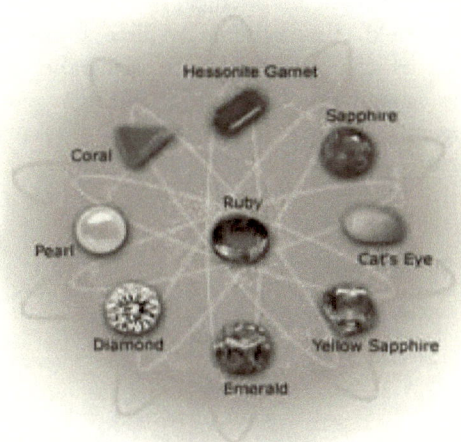

Detecting incoming disease at Aura level in advance is only half the work done. Important part lies in prevention. This can be done by Gems therapy. Gems are concentrated mines of cosmic rays. Gems therapy is vibrational medicine. It is the medicine of future. It is both Holistic and preventive.

There are several reasons for employing gems for healing:-
1. They exhibit pure and single colour.
2. They are exceedingly brilliant with rich contents of rays.
3. They readily and generously release and give out their rays showing no sign of exhaustion.

Ruby, Coral, Moonstone and Cat's Eye are mines of hot cosmic colours. Pearl, Emerald, Diamond, Saphire and Gomed are mines of cold rays.

Ruby being hot, releases hot waves. Combination of Coral and Ruby is very useful for patients suffering from Heart Diseases.

These gems have to be purified, energised and placed at proper positions coinciding with respective endocrine glands for prevention/treatment of diseases.

<u>Gem of treatment</u>

Dr. J.M Shah of Mumbai offers holistic treatment for curing heart problems using a combination of modern science and ancient 'Aura" therapy. According to an ancient medical concept, all living organisms have an "Aura" (energy field) about them. An illness shows an imbalance of colour in the aura which is rectified by wearing the right gem/gems. Dr. Shah has already helped several patients through gem therapy which is cheaper than surgery.

## 3. Dowsing

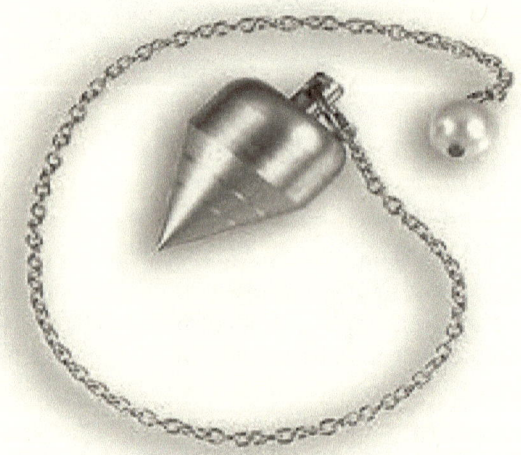

Dowsing is defined as the study of energy field by a person who has electromagnetic ability. This ability is given to us by God as a natural gift or it can be achieved by regular meditation and use of magnetic dresses.

All living and non-living things constantly radiate giving rays of vibrations which are specific like finger prints of each individual.

These rays cause vibrations in the muscle of the dowser and in turn vibrate the pendulum.

### Dowsing is a Vibrational Assesment

Everything in the Universe has a vibration. Each flower, plant, tree, mineral, rock, crystal, or gemstone has its own specific vibration. Each type of cell, organ, system in each living organism also has its own specific vibration. Each thought and emotion has its own vibration. Each sound and color has its own vibration. A Vibrational Assessment is a process where the vibration of a variety of factors is undertaken to identify disharmonious or unbalanced vibrations in the human body and aura. Through dowsing, a Vibrational Assessment read the vibrational energetic signatures within an individual.

Disharmonious or unbalanced vibrations show themselves in many ways including discomfort, dis ease, illness, fatigue, and a variety of different symptoms. When a body is healthy is has a relatively high vibration, and this is reflected through the vibrations of individual cells, organs and systems. When a person is not perfectly healthy the vibrations in the body are lowered. The objective of a Vibrational Assessment is to identify the lower vibrations of various invaders, organs and systems so that remedial action can be taken to raise the vibrations through Choming Essences.

When an individual is not well their body's vibration lowers, the immune system weakens, and manyinvaders enter and stay in a person's body. This includes parasites, worms, bacterial infections, viruses, and different types of fungus. These invaders not only affect the direct functioning of a body, but they also cause other problems since they daily unload many toxins into the human body. Today we are being exposed to many of these invaders on a regular basis. e.g. A simple visit to a hospital can expose you to many infectious bacteria.

### How is A Vibrational Assessment Conducted:

A Vibrational Assessment involves the reading the energetic signature of vibrations which emanate from a variety of factors, by using a pendulum. This is a process whereby an experienced energy dowser connects with the vibrations in and around a physical and auric body and makes an assessment of the presence, and degree of vibration of various factors. Even though many scientists believe that these vibrations do exist, testing methods and equipment have not been devised to measure many of them.

Through distance dowsing, an assessment can be conducted of anyone, anywhere in the world by using the name of an individual. Mary Kurus has conducted many distance assessments to-date and has demonstrated a high degree of accuracy and effectiveness in distance dowsing.

The following is a summary explanation of the specific sections of information contained in a 17 page report of a Vibrational Assessment.

### The Human Aura and Chakras:

The human body is surrounded by energy fields that are called the aura which are layered and interpenetrating. There are many layers to the aura but the ones which I deal with as part of the Vibrational Assessment are the etheric field, which is a three or four inch aura which surrounds the body, fits it like a glove and is an energetic duplicate of the body; the emotional body which is associated with feelings; the mental body which is associated with our ideas and thoughts; and the spiritual body which is associated with spiritual aspects of the individual.

Many factors can affect the various fields of the aura creating holes, breaks in connections, imbalances, and various types of blockages and distortions. Traumas, repressed emotions, negative thought patterns, certain types of emotions, smoking, and the excessive use of drugs and alcohol (including second hand smoke) can affect the vital vibration and effective functioning of the different bodies of the aura. It is a well know fact that smoking and drinking create blockages in auras and chakras.

There are seven major energy centers or chakras within the subtle bodies that draw life giving energy into the physical body, comparable to energy transformers. These are said to resemble whirling vortices of subtle energy. Blockages, holes, tears or other difficulties in the chakras can seriously affect the degree of energy entering the human body and the overall vibration and functioning of the human body.

The Vibrational Assessment will identify the degree of openness of the four auric fields and all seven chakras. This information will be used in support of the overall analysis.

Inner Sound is necessary for intuition for Dowsing

The inner sound is an important facilitator for further development of the nervous system,

The inner energy (kundalini), as described in yoga literature, consists of a stimulus or energy form, originating at the base f the spine (Pc-Muscle) and running along the spine to the brain. The inner energy rising along the spine ideally fills several centers (chakras) also with energy. These centers are along the main nerve strands, which are also being filled with energy. Finally the energy reaches the brain. When sufficient energy reaches the brain, one notices a sound similar to the sound of snake. This is the reason why Indian wise men called this energy snake power. The flow of energy, once it has reached the brain, will continue in a downward mode along the front of the body. This will close the energy circle.

In classical yoga literature, but also in other spiritual systems that deal with life energy and meditation, one perceives an inner tone by removing natural blockages, i.e. during meditation. Can a person perceive this sound in every situation and under all circumstances, we would call this person as having awakened spiritual consciousness. Is the person in union with this inner sound, and can the sound be excited by repeating a certain syllable, the nervous system will be positively activated. This is equivalent to a higher energy level. Besides the activation of inner energy, the perception of the inner sound is a cornerstone of any training in life energy.

### With the Sound of Life Energy to Well-Being and inner Calm:

When the body is totally relaxed and the brain is charged with high energy, one can under ideal conditions, perceive a sound inside the head. It is a moderate level sound like a hissing sound (in the 7 to 9 kHz range), comparable to the chirping sound of the cricket or the sound of an electric motor running at high speed or just like pink noise. In the beginning this ancient sound is very faint, barely noticeable. Unconsciously we remember this sound from the womb, where it was a constant companion while we waited several months to be borne. It reminds us of deep comfort and rest. It was there from the very beginning. All anxieties, all worries and problems came later. Because of that hearing the sound can lead us back to this first experience of a pure untouched condition. Hearing the sound can bring us back to this pure untouched condition. The sound can cause an inner regression leading us back to inner security and openness. Some people fear, when they suddenly hear this sound for the first time, that they suffer from tinnitus, a very unpleasant condition. The perception of the sound is usually, in the middle of the head at the plane of the ears, but sometimes moved to left or right side. As part of our studies with the PcE-Exercises we discovered, that the sound is only noticeable, when the brain is highly charged, when the body is totally relaxed and one is open to the outside. You become conscious of the sound only after a full relaxation of the body muscles, or through the rhythmic contraction of the Pc-Muscle. Chanting, which has nothing do to with breathing or the heart pulse,  brings a feeling of lightness, as if your whole inner being  is being lifted. People who are familiar with meditation or the PcE-Training, add more variation in sounds. The old Germans and Celtics called this sound the "astral sound", or the sound from the other world (autre monde).  Listening to this sound supposedly opens the door to the "autre monde". The Indians call this sound Nadabrahma, the divine sound, or the sound of the snake power kundalini.

If you never consciously perceived your inner sound, you just simply have to search for it. The sound is always there, but gets masked out because of the noise of our daily routine, the anxieties and worries. The best time to hear this sound is just after waking up, or shortly after going to bed, if you are relaxed and listen into the sound. It is most important to relax shoulders, neck, forehead and jaws . Take your time in your search for this inner sound. Once you have heard this sound, it is very easy to reactivate it, in any life situation. It was found that if you are under stress, just imagine this inner sound, and your worries will disappear immediately. We also found that the perception of the inner sound will calm you, when you feel anxious, too excited or even aggressive. One can conclude, that the inner sound is in unison with tranquility and a happy, open mood. If you do not have enough experience with the inner sound, you can lose it as a result of your daily struggles. Pressures, worries, negative attitudes or moods can make the sounds disappear. Whereas the original sound will always be with you are tranquil, relaxed, happy and full of positive energy.

### You should be able to always perceive the inner sound

Utilize the inner sound as your natural feedback system. Before you start with the PcE-meditation, try to perceive the sound in your head. This initially faint and even sound does not change with pulse rate or your blood pressure, can be discovered by listening into it. Once you perceive the sound it means you are totally relaxed and your head is free. This enables you to receive more energy from within anf from outside. In practice this means, that you listen into yourself, until you perceive the sound and hold on to it, by softly concentrating on it. If the sound level increases, you are doing fine, but if the sound level decreases again or disappears, it means you are tensing up. The tensions are mostly muscular in nature and occur in shoulders, neck and forehead. Try to control these muscles and remove the blockages. It was found helpful, to tighten these muscles even more for just a few seconds, and the relax them again with rocking motions and head circling. Once you are relaxed again, listen into yourself and hold on to the inner sound. The sound should become stronger and easier to perceive. Practice the activation for several weeks, and you should be able to hear the sound in noise or when under stress, whenever you desire. This is now your natural feedback system, which is available to you at any time. You can always check, what your present state is and determine, if you are under stress, when the sound can not be perceived. If you suppress your inner sound, you subject yourself to the rhythms of life with its worries, pressures and anxieties. Check several times during the day, if you perceive the inner sound, and within a short time, you have the capacity to restore inner calm and tranquility at will.

**Where and how does the inner sound originate?**

How this sound originates is still very unclear. One thing we do know is, that the sound is perceived in the center of the temple bones and is also generated there. This increases the energy flow in that part of the brain and distributors to the rest of the brain. The discovery of the PcE effect and the potential measurements with the PcE-Trainer revealed to us, that as soon as the inner sound is perceived, the centers of the temples become totally transparent and enables the person to tap into higher consciousness. We were totally fascinated in our research of life energy when we discovered, that the inner sound leads to a higher activation of energy.

The temples for some time now have become a preferred research topic with many neurologists and biologists, for a good reason. Anybody who is interested in extraordinary capacities and perceptions, needs to study the function of the temples.

At the end of the sixties the South- African Gordon Nelson recorded EEG signals from trance subjects and noticed special EEG temples. It was later found, that electric discharge in the temples can alter the way information is perceived, enabling the person to become conscious of perceptions that would normally go right into the unconscious without ever being recognized.

EEG-Research of Qigong-Masters with simultaneous PET scans of regional blood flow in the brain showed also, that during Qigong the temples and the Hippocampus (these two brain areas work together) were highly activated, whereas the rest of the brain remained quiet. Our lab test revealed, that as soon as one increases the UL-potentials of the temples with biofeedback (focus), people experience extrasensory perception. The inner sound is just one of the possibilities, to consciously activate the temples in a controlled manner. This means: if you can not only further increase your inner energy, but also during your meditation remove any barriers or filters to higher perceptions.

**Perception of the inner Sound**

**What is the mechanism of increased energy when we hear the inner sound?**

We have to observe the function of our sense organs, especially the hearing, more closely.

The brain receives electrical potentials through the action (stimuli) of all sensory organs.

This means that every sensory organ generates a flow of energy to the brain (certain sections of the brain) which charges the brain.

The proven strongest energy producer is our hearing and the connected brain area. The ears with 90% of the energy production of all sensory organs to the cortex is the most important. This is mostly due to the reception of higher frequencies (4000 to 8000 Hz and higher). The perception of these higher frequencies generates a high rate of impulses, which charge the brain (mainly the temples and the frontal lobes). This can be verified with ULP measurements of these areas with the PcE-Trainer.

These brain charges mean: awakened consciousness, better thinking and learning, positive life attitude, better memory, more will-power. In one word: more vitality, creativity and enjoyment of life.

For the benefit of your meditation, you can download a recording of an inner sound for listening. We recommend that you play the sound during meditation. If you listen to it more frequently, it will be easy for you to invoke the sound through mere imagination and remembrance

4. Prayers

1) Prayer is a ultimate tool of asking help from divine power.

2) While praying man connects his own soul power to the supreme soul unknowingly.

3) It is proved that if you pray on exact time every day without fail, your prayers are answered effectively.

4) Regular prayer helps the human to clean his negative energies.

## Prayer Timings for Health, Wealth and Happiness

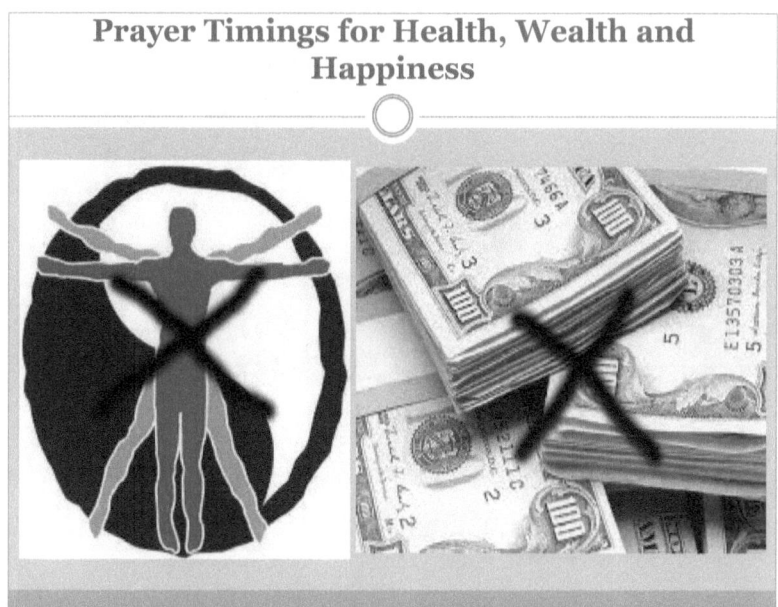

## Meaning of Atmosphere

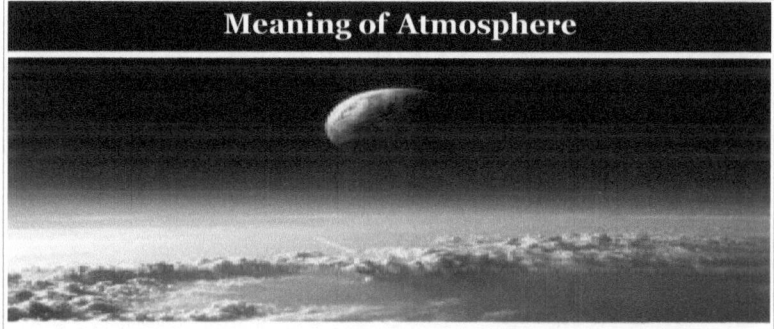

Dictionary meaning of Atmosphere is Gasses surrounding earth and other planets. It is quiet in normal course.

## Atmosphere Changes

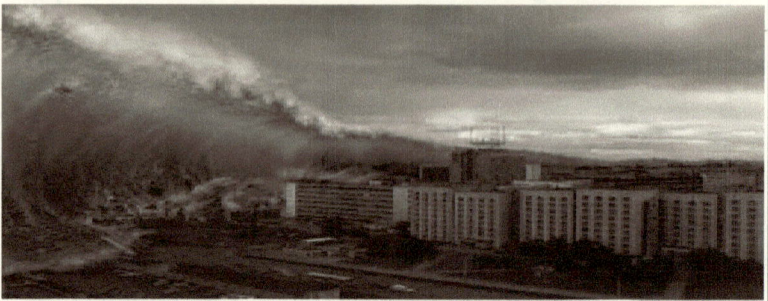

As per religious Books major Disturbances in atmosphere take place 72 min before sunrise, at sunrise, at midday & at sunset. Dark Energy is generated at these times and enters our Aura. .

# Sickness

**Unhappiness can come in the form of sickness in our physical body, like Heart problems, breathing problems & even cancer.**

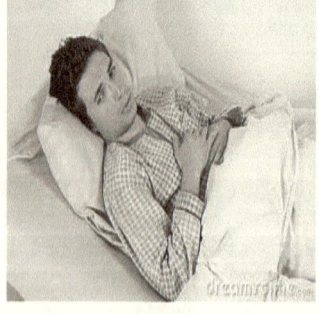

# Financial Loss

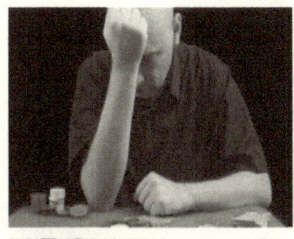

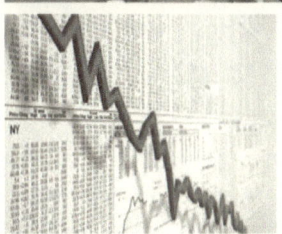

Dark energy also disturbs our prosperity and brings financial loss. It also disturbs our family and social life.

# J ain prayers

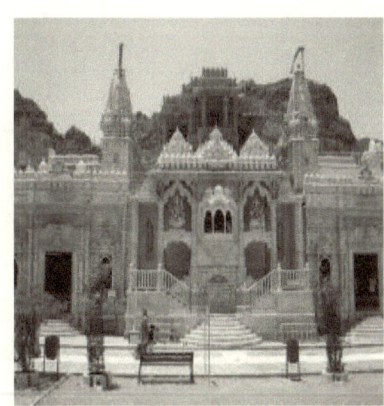

*According to jain religion seven times prayers in a day keeps us healthy, wealthy & prosperous. These are the timings when there is disturbance in Atmosphere resulting in generation of dark energy.*

# Islamic namaj

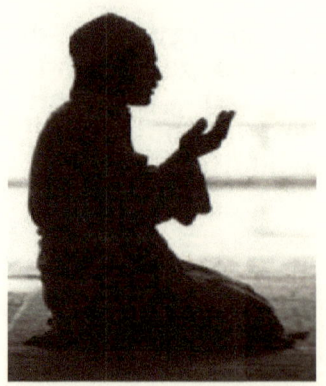

**According to islam religion also there are seven times of prayers (namaj).**

## Agnihotra

Many people in 62 countries of the world perform agnihotra at specific time of sunrise and sunset. According to a survey, persons performing agnihotra regularly are healthy wealthy and prosperous.

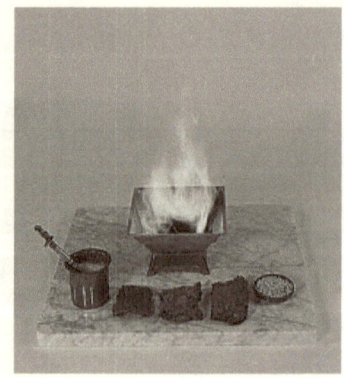

# Timing of prayers

- Prayer timings mentioned in religious books are very important because these are the times when dark energy is generated in the atmosphere.

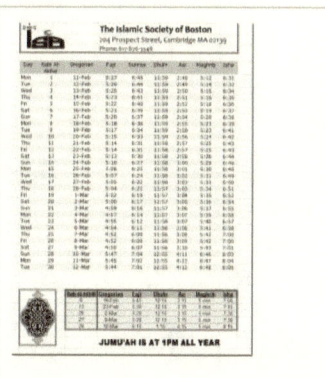

# How to remain Healthy, Happy and Prosperous.

BY DR.J.M.SHAH

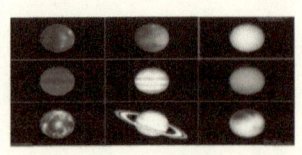
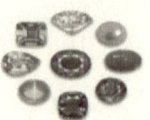

IT IS DIFFICULT TO FIND A PERSON ON EARTH WHO
DOES NOT WANT TO BE HEALTHY AND HAPPY.

AS PER ASTROLOGICAL PRINCIPLES HEALTH AND
HAPPINESS COME TO US ONLY WHEN NINE
PLANETS ARE FAVORABLE TO US.

THIS IS POSSIBLE WITH THE HELP OF GEMSTONES.

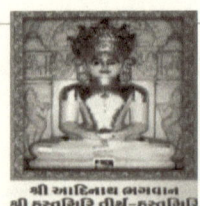

श्री આदिनાथ ભગવાન
श्री हस्तगिरि तीर्थ-हस्तगिरि

DIVINE ENERGY OF GOD CAN BE
CONSIDERED AS SUM TOTAL OF
ENERGIES OF NINE PLANETS.
THESE PLANETS GOVERN OUR
LIFE FROM THE TIME WE ARE
BORNED TILL THE TIME WE DIE.

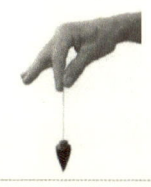

## Dowsing

DURING OUR LIFE CYCLE, SOME PLANETS ARE FAVORABLE TO US AT SPECIFIC TIMES AND UNFAVORABLE AT OTHER TIMES. WHEN NINE PLANETS ARE FAVORABLE WE ARE HAPPY, HEALTHY AND PROSPEROUS. WHEN NOT HEATH PROBLEMS, FINANCE PROBLEMS & SOCIAL PROBLEMS CROP UP.

WITH THE HELP OF GEMSTONES, IT IS POSSIBLE TO KEEP PLANETS FAVORABLE TO US.

A SPIRITUAL DOWSER CAN FIND REQUIRED GEMSTONES TO GIVE US HAPPINESS IN FAMILY, SOCIETY, PERSONAL MATTERS, BUSINESS AND OUR HEALTH.

## Bio-Well Camera

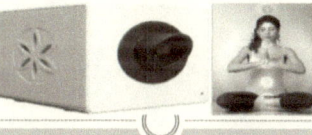

GEMSTONES MAKE TWELVE HOUSES OF OUR HOROSCOPE FAVORABLE TO US.
WITH THE HELP OF BIO-WELL CAMERA WE CAN SEE THE RESULT OF GEMSTONES BY TAKING PRE AND POST AURA PHOTOGRAPHY.

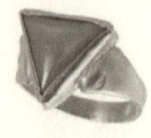 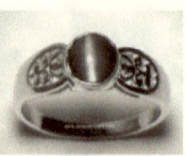

## Gemstones

**REPORT AFTER WEARING 2 GEMSTONES
CORAL AND CATSEYE.**

**ENERGY FIELD :- 67 JOULES**

**CHAKRAS POSITION
CHAKRA JOULES:-    5 JOULES .
ALL CHAKRAS ALIGNED.**

**DISEASES :-  NOT SHOWING DISEASES**

Conclusion

To remain Happy and Healthy, use of required Gemstones play very vital part. They can be found by a spiritual Dowser.

Correctness of Gemstones can be verified by Aura Photography by Bio-Well Camera.

Effect of Gemstones can be supported by offering prayers at specific times available in internet under "Prayer Timings". Alternatively, morning and evening Agnihotra can be performed as per details available in internet.

**Dr. J.M.Shah & Dr. Korotkov**

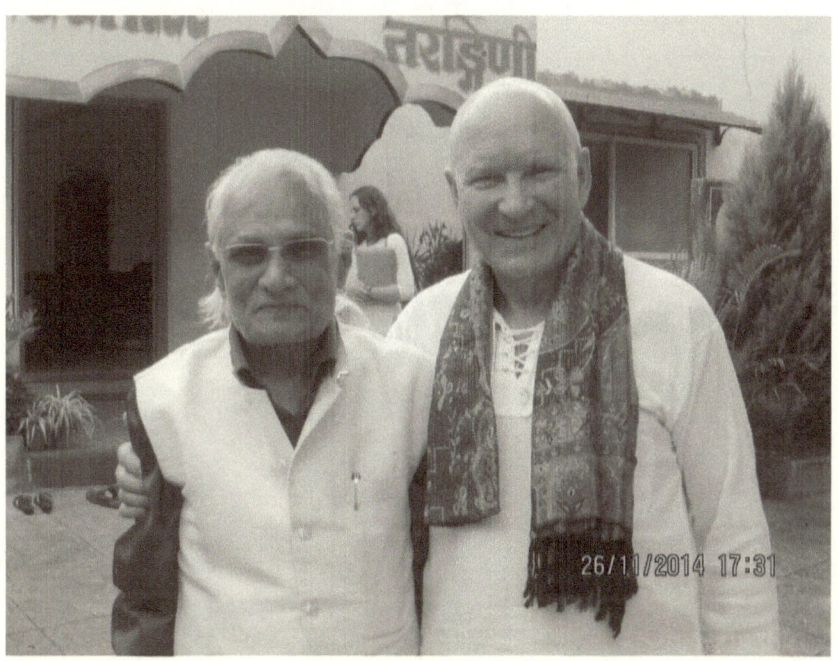

**Video Links:-**

1) **6min Aura Photography video link**
   https://youtu.be/KVeWINEMrVE

   2) **Press conference video link**
   https://youtu.be/QAz41xebq_U

3) **Introducing Bio-Well video link**
   https://youtu.be/pTjyEwYRkF4
   4) **Kirlian Photography Dr. J.M. Shah video link**
   https://youtu.be/mXERXcKA7UE

   5) **Hon. Prime Minister Narendra Modi Ji video link**
   https://youtu.be/01Z5YCNOupw

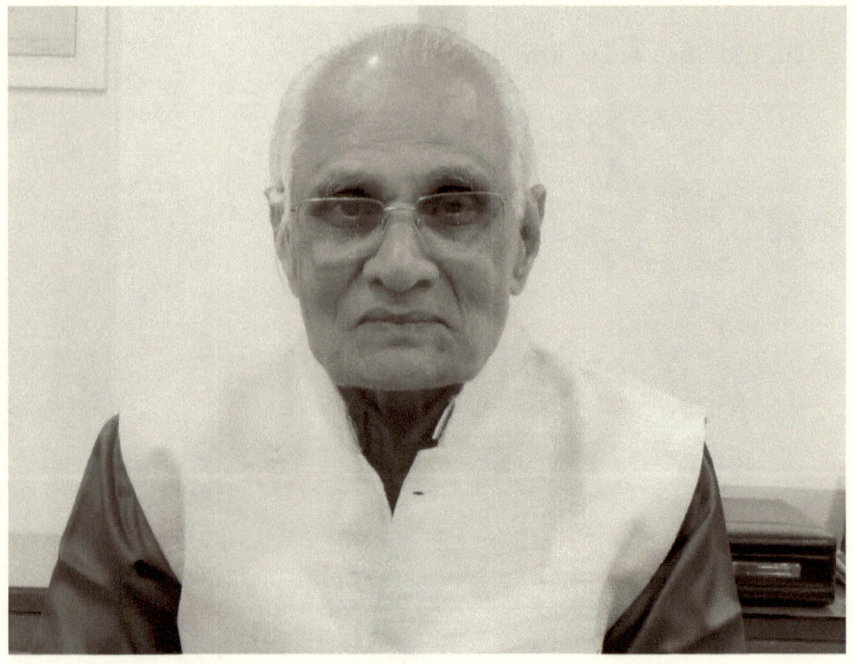

**Dr. Jashvant Shah**

Hi, my name is Jashvant and I am the Chairman & Managing Director of SURU Group of Companies.

www.hrjsurgicals.com
www.suruchemical.co.in
www.suru.com

I am Pharmacy graduate from Gujarat University of 1962 batch. I worked for a Pharmaceutical company manufacturing injections for 15 years.

I started my own business SURU Chemical & Pharmaceuticals Pvt Ltd in 1973 as a Small Scale Unit for manufacturing Lanolin, a raw material for Pharmaceuticals & Cosmetics.
www.suruchemical.co.in
After 3 years I started other 2 companies HRJ Surgicals and SURU International Pvt Ltd for manufacturing disposable surgical devices. SURU International is an Export Oriented Unit in Dahanu, Maharashtra State with international clients.

Our group company received Top Exporter Award from PHARMEXCIL in 1985 and another company received SSI Award from the hands of Vice President of India in the same year.

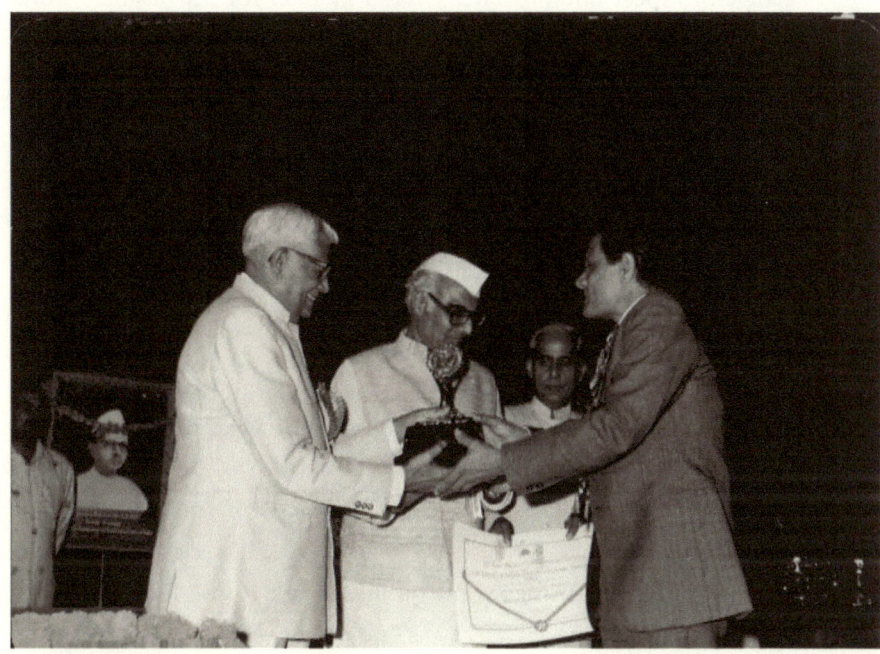

In this year our group company received sponsorship for 45 days tour from United Nations for business development in America and Canada.

Our group company also received several Safety Awards.

We started participating in Medica Trade Fair in Germany every year from 1993 after getting training from Netherlands Govt. for business.

**MY HOBBY :**

In 1992 I read an article in Times of India about conference in Kerala on Aura Photography. In the article it was also mentioned that by Aura Photography it was possible to see full body health problem, at present as well as 4 – 6 months in future.

I was interested in this subject as it was connected with Health.

At this time my mother was 90 years old and had age related problems and this was one of the reasons for my interest. It was very difficult to take her to pathology laboratory for blood test report, X ray report, ECG etc. Aura photograph would avoid all this hassles.

I happen to meet one Mr. Henry Bawa in 1993 for my business work. He was wearing gemstones on his body at various places on hand with a cello tape. I enquired about this that generally gemstones are worn as rings and pendant, why you have placed on various places on hands. He explained to me that during medication he gets divine messages about healing powers of precious gemstones. For example gemstone of Sun is Ruby and that of Mars is Coral. Both are hot in nature. On keeping them on the area of hearts they energize the heart by increasing it subtle energy. I worked in India on about 15 patients with heart problems and received good results. That time I had Black and White Aura camera, which I used to see treatment results by Pre and Post treatment Aura Photography.

I received my PhD degree in this year from Open International University for complementary medicine for work on heart problems.

My work on Gemstone Therapy was recorded in Limca Book of World Record in 1997.

In this year I visited Russia for my business work.

Incidentally at that time there was a seminar on Aura Photography by GDV Aura Camera inventor *Dr. Konstantin Korotkov*. Dr. Korotkov invited me to present my work on Gem Stone Therapy in the seminar.

Dr. Korotkov also arranged for joint case study on heart patient in Pokrovskaya Hospital in St. Petersburg, Russia. His team took pre and post treatment aura photograph of Russian heart patients. I gave treatment by Gem Stone therapy.

11 out of 13 patient got good results. My treatment lasted for 7 days.

Pokrovskaya hospital Dean prepared a report on the project and handed over this report to Indian Ambassador in St. Petersburg, Russia.

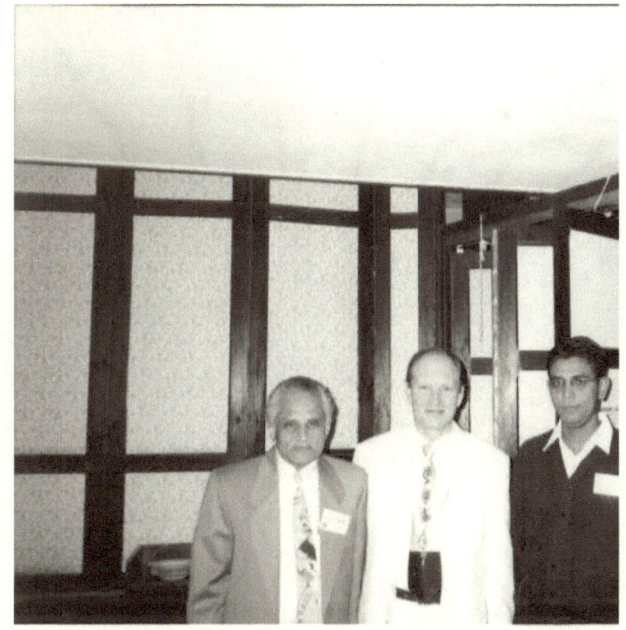

**Dr J M Shah with Dr Korotkov**

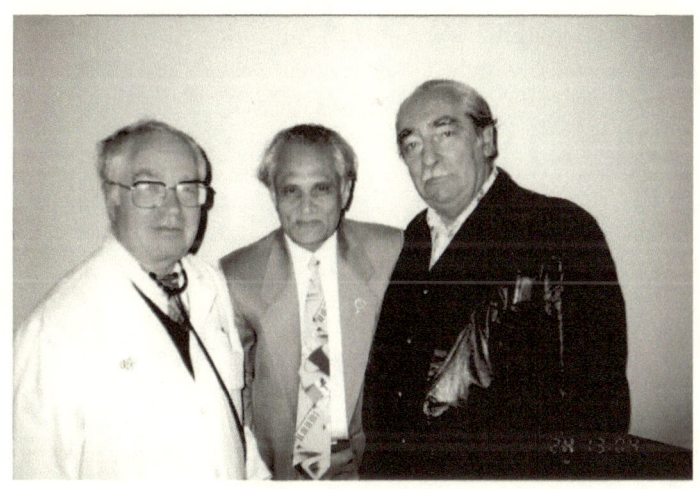

**Dr. J.M. Shah with Dr. Kukuyi**

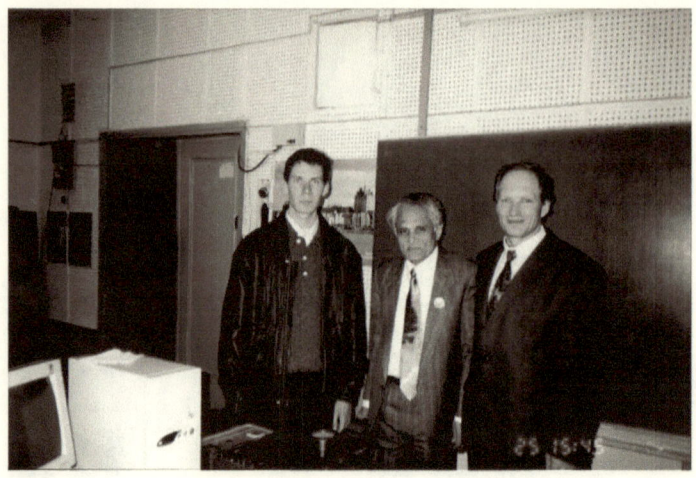

**Dr J M Shah in Russian Lab**

I started Kirlian photography centre in 2014 for Aura Photography to know health problems at present as well as in future. In this year we received distributorship from Dr. Korotkov for Bio Well Aura Camera for India.

We are present in social media:

  Website:  www.jmshah.com

  https://www.facebook.com/aura.photography.jms?ref=hl

  https://www.linkedin.com/profile/public-profile-settings?trk=prof-edit-edit-public_profile

  https://twitter.com/AuraPhotograph

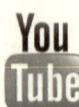  https://www.youtube.com/watch?v=C_ern1w7dA4

# 2

## ANYONE CAN BE A LEADER!
### *(AND WHEN WE CHOOSE TO LEAD...ANYTHING IS POSSIBLE.)*

#### - BY DAVID SPUNGIN, FOUNDER & PRINCIPAL CONSULTANT, THE LEADER GROWTH GROUP, LLC.

It was a hot summer day in 2003 and our small team of soldiers was preparing to leave our base camp in Baghdad, Iraq for another routine re-supply mission. We had done many such missions over the past few months and in my often-monotonous role as a staff officer supporting combat operations, I had come to enjoy these opportunities to get "outside the wire" and interact with the local populace. However, this day was to be a little different. Donning our bulletproof body armor, Kevlar helmets, and tactical vests carrying extra ammunition, everyone was sweating profusely under the equipment's weight. With our pre-mission checks completed we lined up our convoy of vehicles to exit the base camp, but were abruptly stopped at the gate by the guard on duty. Showing me a picture of what looked to be an artillery shell buried in the ground with wires coming out of it, he explained that this was our enemy's new weapon of choice and that we needed to be on the lookout. Today we know this to be an I.E.D. (Improvised Explosive Device) and people are well aware of their lethality, yet at the time, they were a brand new weapon on the battlefield and mostly unheard of.

As we cruised swiftly on the highway to our destination, I remember the air being so hot that day; it felt as if someone was holding a hair dryer directly in your face! Soon though, we arrived at the Baghdad marketplace and began our familiar pattern of bargaining with our preferred merchants. Everything was going just as planned and, with our new supplies loaded in our vehicles, we set back out for base camp without incident. Then suddenly, there was an extremely loud BOOM! It was a massive explosion that knocked me forward in my seat. Immediately I recalled the I.E.D. briefing we'd received and my heart sank as the reality of the situation set in. Grabbing the radio, I contacted our other team members and requested a status report. Everyone checked-in fine and we slowed to the side of the road to further assess the situation. As we surveyed the scene around us, it became apparent that another convoy had been hit on the other side of the highway. The enemy had likely tried to get a "two for one" and hit us both simultaneously as our convoys were within a few feet of one another at the time of the explosion. Then I noticed the burning U.S. vehicle on the other side of the road. We had to do something, but what? None of us were trained on how to react to an I.E.D., and in fact, the only thing we did know was not to move towards an attack as there were often multiple bombs waiting for others who rushed to help. A decision had to be made and as the ranking officer in our convoy, I needed to provide some direction quickly.

After conferring with my senior non-commissioned officers, we made the call to dismount our vehicles and cross the road to provide assistance to the other convoy. By the time we arrived on the scene, other soldiers had already pulled the crew members out of the burning vehicle and were giving them medical attention. I thought there must be some other way we could still help and that's when we noticed the large group of people walking towards us. Local residents were curious as to what had happened and were now spontaneously circling us and the wounded soldiers. Immediately, I gave the order to secure the area and our team began the difficult task of crowd control. We moved the now slightly hostile crowd back from the scene and created a semi-circle around the damaged vehicle with our backs to the highway. Then, perhaps due to our difficulty in communicating and the overall stress of the situation, tempers began to flare up. Groups within the crowd were now yelling at our guys and, for the first time in our deployment, I saw confused and scared U.S. soldiers brandishing their weapons with truly hostile intentions. What's worse, I noticed that we were also standing very close to a highway overpass. Those that study military history know that he who holds the high ground wins. If the enemy who detonated this I.E.D. were to simply walk onto that overpass, they would have open fields of fire onto all of us. It was clear that my recent decisions had put us all into a bad situation and something had to be done about it immediately.

Without further hesitation, I began to work with my non-commissioned officers to pull a few soldiers off our perimeter in order to establish nearside and far-side security on the overpass. It was relieving to see our guys take their newly elevated positions, as I knew they could now see down onto the crowd and identify any potential problems. Satisfied we were now well positioned, I began to focus on the emotional aspects of the situation at hand. Walking our perimeter and checking in with each soldier, I did my best to ease their tension and calm down any hostilities with the crowd. We were all pretty scared, not necessarily of the immediate danger to us personally, but more fearful of the potential for escalating violence. Even for a trained soldier, the possibility of actually having to commit an act of violence against another human at point blank range can be an unsettling experience. Thankfully, I was working alongside a group of extraordinary cavalrymen who were all quite competent and who wholeheartedly trusted one another. Everyone did an amazing job of both keeping the crowd at bay and tempering their emotions. Within 20 minutes or so, the injured soldiers were evacuated and help arrived to assist us. We then collapsed our perimeter and headed back to our vehicles. We had avoided a potentially disastrous situation and returned safely without further incident.

Why was our team effective in handling this volatile and ambiguous challenge? One might point to any number of reasons ranging from superior training to dumb luck. However, I offer that the key ingredient to our success that day is the same as what makes any great team successful — leadership. Not just my leadership, but also the leadership exhibited by every non-commissioned officer and soldier on our team that day. We succeeded because we operated within a true culture of leadership where everyone was expected to execute their roles well and lead themselves first. Ultimately, this is a story of decisiveness, situational awareness, resiliency, adaptability, initiative, communication, teamwork, self-management, accountability, and self-less service. In essence, it is a story of how leadership delivers success. Yet, none of us in this story were born with a divine understanding of how these characteristics might enable our success or enhance our ability to lead. No, instead we had all been taught leadership over time through the Army's culture and given many opportunities to practice these principles. The result is that when we needed it most, leadership simply happened.

I share this story with you because it is a good illustration of how and why I founded a leader development company focused on transforming managers into truly inspiring leaders. After 20 plus years of personally leading teams and formally studying leader development, such experiences have allowed me to draw a few important conclusions about leadership. It's through these conclusions that I was ultimately inspired to do this work and I would like to share them with you.

To begin, I believe that leaders are made not born. Anyone can learn to be a leader and that's because leadership is an activity, not a position. Many often mistake their boss as their "leader," yet leadership has nothing to do with title or authority and everything to do with the choices an individual makes. When a person chooses to exhibit leadership behaviors, he or she increases their ability to influence others. Moreover, when a person begins to truly embody these behaviors, that is, they behave like a leader because that is simply who they have become, they cannot fail but to inspire others to greatness! This was a particularly important realization for me as a leader development professional because I came to understand that leadership is a choice that we all have available to us. Either you choose leadership behaviors and activities that inspire others or you don't. This simple truth is what determines the leader from the non-leader.

Another key conclusion I have drawn has to do with where leadership is exercised within an organization. For over a century now, the top-down, pyramidal, command and control style of exercising leadership has dominated our corporate hierarchies. While many intuitively recognize that monopolizing power at the top is an undesirable practice, this is what we are most familiar with. We often self-perpetuate the pains of these bureaucratic models because it's comfortable. Yet, time and again, I've found that organizations that foster a culture of leadership throughout the entire organization are the most effective. You might be wondering how a person with such a military heavy background could possibly understand anything other than a command and control style of leadership. If you are making that assumption, you couldn't be farther from the truth. In fact, the

U.S. military is the largest, most empowered organization in the world. Leadership is taught at all levels and in the absence of direct orders, the lowest private is trusted to make bold decisions that might affect the lives of many. Imagine what could happen if your organization operated like this as well. Are there any limits to the possibilities that you might collectively achieve together? This very thought is what drives me every day. I believe there is so much untapped leadership potential that is just waiting to be discovered.

So why then have we not made greater strides in debunking these leadership myths and gotten better at creating leaders at all levels of the modern organization? Well, the challenges are many. For one, leadership is an art that can only be developed over time and the best way to learn leadership is by 1) being exposed to leadership, 2) reflecting upon it, and 3) practicing it through direct experience. With this in mind, who in our organization is going to do this important work of teaching leadership? Ideally, our manager would also be a fine leader who had the time and expertise to teach us leadership skills. Yet, the modern manager is an extremely busy and overtaxed individual. Then, even if they are excellent leaders and teachers themselves, ensuring operational excellence often trumps mentoring on their list of never-ending priorities. So then, realistically, what happens? Organizations get in the habit of simply promoting people based on their technical competence rather than their leadership acumen. The thought is that leadership will be learned on the job, but leadership doesn't just happen with promotion! Too often the result is a technically competent but mediocre leader who creates places where people feel unappreciated, bored, apathetic, and without purpose. Over time this leads to average performance results at best which no company can sustain over time in a highly competitive, globalized marketplace.

These very real challenges are ultimately why I created The Leader Growth Group, LLC. Too much potential has been wasted for far too long, and I've witnessed how a sustained leader development program can help reverse this trend. Yet, not all training and coaching is the same and there are some important distinctions to consider when choosing to grow your leadership talent. First, many programs teach "about" leadership and, while that will help one to understand what leadership is, it rarely translates into application of that knowledge. Bridging this "knowing-doing gap" is always a challenge and this is why experiencing leadership firsthand is often the best teacher. In all of my programs, I seek to create the conditions for people to teach themselves leadership. I incorporate experiential activities to help ground important lessons and work to take the complexity out of leadership by making it simple and relatable. People best learn leadership when training or coaching is realistic, practical, and a good balance of experiencing significant challenge and unwavering support.

I have also come to learn that creating these conditions for learning leadership is truly an art form. Thus, one should consider the quality of the trainers/coaches that you select to do this work. It can be challenging to find a person who both understands leadership firsthand through their own experiences and is adept at teaching leadership to others. I believe this is my forte. I feel as if I have a unique ability to connect with a wide range of audiences, from teaching front-line workers with no formal leadership experience to coaching top executives. This is because I embody what I teach. People learn leadership not just through what I say, but also through the entirety of the experience. They recognize that I am passionate about helping them to increase their self-awareness and self-management capacity. They notice how I thrive in facilitating discussion about difficult conversations that leaders and teams might not otherwise engage in. They identify with how I love turning the light on in individuals, helping them to see their potential and ability to serve others.

Know that your leadership is needed in this world! If my message of leadership or how to develop leaders resonates with you, I invite you to connect with me personally via the contact information provided at the end of this chapter. I would also like to extend you a gift. Please log onto http://ebook.leadergrowthgroup.com/actionableleadership to get a free copy of my "Actionable! Leadership" eBook and learn how to develop your inspirational ability, motivate teams, and achieve extraordinary results. This eBook captures many of my most important leader development insights from twenty plus years of coaching and training leaders. It is designed to help leaders at all levels identify areas for growth and discover tangible ways to improve their leadership abilities. I welcome the opportunity to learn more about you and your organization, and wish you much success in reaching your full leadership potential!

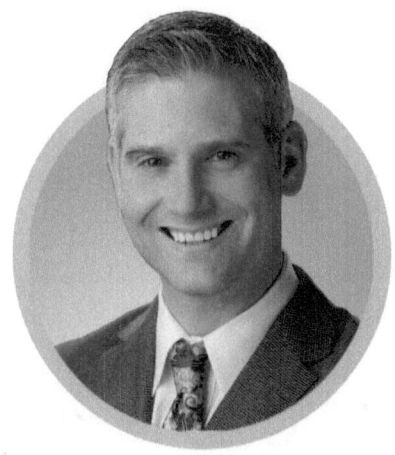

## David Spungin

David is a Corporate Trainer, Speaker, and Executive Coach focused on transforming managers into high performing leaders. He holds a degree in Leadership Development from the United States Military Academy at West Point, a Master of Science in Organization Development from American University, and has completed advanced leadership studies at Harvard University. A U.S. Army combat veteran with corporate leadership experience, he now consults to primarily Fortune 500 companies. He is recognized for his ability to quickly assess an organization's culture, develop creative learning designs, and facilitate highly engaging training events. David holds expertise in the MBTI, DiSC, EQ-i 2.0 and PMAI behavioral assessments, as well as in non-verbal (somatic) communication. Additionally, he is an International Coaching Federation (ICF) certified coach.

### Specialties

Customized and Experiential Leadership Training that Delivers Results
Leadership Coaching for Managers, Directors, & Executives
Dynamic Speaking Engagements that Inspire & Motivate Teams
Distance/Blended Leader Development Training Solutions & Customized Webinars
Non-Verbal Communication & Developing Executive Presence
Building Team Cohesiveness & Effectiveness
Organizational Culture Assessment & Transformation Initiatives

Generating Greater Emotional Intelligence
Fostering Employee Retention & Engagement

**Contact Information**

Email David directly at dspungin@leadergrowthgroup.com or phone him at +1.720.485.5687

Visit the Leader Growth Group, LLC. Website at www.leadergrowthgroup.com

Follow David's blog at http://davidspungin.com/

Connect with David on LinkedIn at https://www.linkedin.com/in/davidspungin

Follow David on Twitter at https://twitter.com/davidspungin

Follow the Leader Growth Group on Facebook at https://www.facebook.com/leadergrowthgroup

# 3

## DREAM, GROW AND TEAM WORK
### LEADERSHIP KEYS TO SUCCESS AND LIVING YOUR LIFE SECRET FROM YOUR HEART

- BY XESCO ESPAR, AUTHOR, SPEAKER, INTUITIVE LIFE COACH.

In our innermost being, we all know that we live three parallel lives: the private life, the public life and the secret life. Although we spend most of our time between the first two, it is inside the third where our greatest dreams are forged.

The secret life is based on three principles: first, *have the courage to dream* that anything is possible; see you future, imagine it as vividly as possible. Second, learn, grow and *become someone who deserves that dream*, and finally if at the end the task is that big, *use the power of teamwork* to achieve your dream.

Here's how I see personal leadership to live life from your heart.


## MY STORY

My life has always been related to sport and high personal performance.

As a kid, I started playing team-handball because in my school sport was a fundamental part of the education. To be honest, I was taller and stronger than talented.

Our school team had considerable success. This allowed me to enter the FC Barcelona as a young player. I even got to play in the professional team. But there were some differences between the coach and I, regarding my exact position in the team. I thought it was on the court and he always decided it was on the bench. So I thought that if I have to stay on the bench, at least I'd rather be the boss. So I retired as a player at 22 years and became a sport coach.

This decision actually allowed me to anticipate nearly 10 years in life. Most coaches who were players retire at age 32 or 34 instead. but for me, at 22 I started to prepare myself as a coach so one day I could coach a professional team.

When I started coaching young players, I begun working for a junior team. They didn't get the National Championship for the last ten years since, neither I did in the first year. Too much concerned about winning, I focused on achieving more wins than working to train and develop the players.

At the end of the first year, when I was doing my personal evaluation I realized that instead of playing to win, we better trained to grow and create professional players (which is more difficult than winning). That would mean working not only for improving young players' career, but the chances of winning the championship would increase immediately!

With that in mind, we doubled our training schedule and design a plan to work with weights, to maximize the strength of the new players. Despite not having the permission of the directors, I convinced the cleaning man to let us enter the gym in exchange for us to clean the gym before leaving.

Over the next five years we conquered not only 4 national championships, but also send more than 10 players into the professional world. In its medium-term future these players won the European Champions League as professional players on several occasions, even got to reach the World Championship in 2005 with the Spanish national team.

In 1997 and after 12 years coaching young players my desire changed into training professional players. However, before me another opportunity arose.

I was offered to participate in the professional team as and assistant, and take care of the physical coaching part of the program. I accepted. My idea was to start as assistant but to become one day the head coach of that team.

The early years with my team were tremendously successful. Within 5 consecutive years we won the European Championship and the Spanish league. We became a legend in European Tam Handball.

However, on the year 2000 a political law changed in Spain and the possibilities for building houses increased exponentially. Immediately local governments (collecting a lot more taxes because of buildings) and building companies had a lot of money that invested in handball teams in cities where there football teams were not strong.

That's why teams from Valladolid, Leon and especially Pamplona and Ciudad Real raised their budgets to compete with us, they signed several of our best players and we stop winning.

I spent these seven years not only as Athletic Trainer, but learning about the most successful methodologies on human performance.

During those years, there was another team in the world also very successful: the Swedish National team. In a conversation with his coach I could detect the two qualities necessary to be a championship team, which later would determine one of my main theories about human performance. Having a champion team is based on two main pillars: 1/ an exhaustive and comprehensive description of team game plan and 2/ a high sense of responsibility and self-discipline hold by all team members.

At the end of the 2003-04 season and after four years in which no major titles the coach decided to retire.

I have to say that there was no chance for me to become the head coach because I was seen just as the Athletic Trainer. *But in life there are times when you have to take charge of your own way*, so I asked for an appointment with the president of the Club to explain my reasons for being coach. Although initially he only gave me 10 minutes the meeting was extended for an hour and when the meeting was over I was selected as the coach the following year.

In my first year as head coach, the team won the European Champions League. In the second year we won the Spanish National Championship.

The third year was a difficult year. At a request of the president of the club I accepted the collaboration on the team of a former player who did not want me to be the coach. After a few weeks had convinced many members that it would be better to change coach. Despite these difficulties, that year we get to win the King's Cup, another big tournament in Spain.

At the end of the year, despite having renewed the contract just three months before, I was told that there would be a change in coaching the team next year.

So at age 47 I decided to leave the sport world and make a jump to nowhere.

Nowhere?

No. Not really. I decided I was going to find a way to reach a larger part of society with my knowledge about high performance and on this way, monetize all that knowledge.

I decided that instead of training to 20 athletes, was going to train thousands of people.

The first step was to write a book: *Play from your heart*, explaining my experiences and my particular angle to look at life during the past 10 years. This book allowed me to transition from someone unknown to most people, to someone who was asked for autographs down the street.

My philosophy is simple: First, you dream what you want. Never set easy targets! Looking objectives that require you to give the best of yourself, so you have to use all your resources and you will develop safely.

Second, pay the price to grow until you deserve the goal you have set.

And third, if this goal is as big as it should be, it is essential to create a support team. You just do not get it so you will need to lean on a team. If that team gets to live by the values of a real team, then get the magic of synergy that makes $1 + 1 = 3$

I thought I was more than a sport coach. I had prepared both in the years that I was capable of any company. That's what gives you confidence. When you think about the things that have left you well.

I returned to teach at the University. It is great to teach youn people because I feel teaching young students rejuvenates me too.

And for the rest of my professional life I designed four focal points to re-start my own business.

First I started working with senior and middle managers of large corporations. I teach them what is the exact the role that talent and motivation play, so they can access themselves to their best personal and professional performance and help and inspire their employees to achieve its best level as well.

Second, I also work with sales forces and train them as high performance players so they can improve their performance habits and sustainably achieve their best results each month without being at the expense of how customers or market behave.

Third, I'm currently working with coaches and professional athletes to help them to attain their maximum performance possible. They develop their talent and motivation in pursuit of excellence in their participation in Olympic Games, National Leagues and International Competitions.

And finally, I work with people who want to be extraordinary in their life but still give too much power to the environment. I help them reclaim and find their own power, to analyze the main obstacles they face, to progress and grow to deserve the greatest success they can imagine.

## MY TAKEAWAYS

**Personal performance: Talent times passion**

Personal performance is the result of a simple but powerful equation: talent x passion.

Talent is the quality factor of the equation. Talent is not only represents the amount of technical skills we possess, but should also include our ability to use these techniques in challenging environments. Expressing you talent when things are easy is not hard. The problem appears when you should do that in difficult times.

And finally there's a third component regarding talent: talent should also include the ability to anticipate events, so you can act proactively and lead your field.

The talent is irreplaceable and should always be developed to its best. When the maximum is reached then look for to redefine it and continue growing. Developing your talent is a mission of a lifetime.

The other part of the equation is the passion we feel for our work. The passion for doing things determines the amount of talent that we use every day.

**Dream! The bright part of success**

All my life I dreamed of being a professional coach. I firmly believe that what we dream is always the first step to get something big in life.

Since our childhood we dream in our future. As years pass by the world takes charge and decides for us. Immerse into a cloud of mediocrity, we tend to forget our dreams and too often decide to lower our goals so people around us don't feel insecure.

Nothing irritates me more.

If one thing I've learned is that we must dream. Setting bold goals for our future brings passion to our life! Dreaming of a better spectacular future will wake you up every day with unlimited energy.

When dreaming imagine a perfect future. Include your family, your friends, your colleagues ... Imagine how you should grow to achieve that dream and visualize yourself acquiring unexpected skills that make you the special person who can give life a lot more than others expect.

Sometimes society seeks to stop our dreams and do not call "delusional" for believing that we can achieve any goal. It says that if we are too lofty goals, and at the end we are not going to get, we will not disappoint and the result may be worse. These goals should be achievable.

Never let your present the results influence your goals!

To know if a goal is good for you, when you put a target your legs should tremble and wonder if you have chosen your or it is the goal that chose you.

There are no impossible goals, just in case there are audacious deadlines.

### Grow! The forgotten side of success

I have seen a lot of people to let go of their dreams because they don't know that dreams are deserved, not only pursued.

The secret to having an amazing life is to be willing to pay the price to grow to deserve it.

No goal is too high if you are willing to pay the price to grow. And when we grow, we have a powerful ally who we usually take as an enemy. I mean obstacles.

Obstacles are actually gifts that come from your dreams. Your objectives communicate with you through obstacles. They will hint and tell you who you must become in order to deserve what you want.

Far from paralyzing us, obstacles should help us to raise... what do I need to still have to overcome this obstacle? Rather than immobilize us obstacles should help us to grow.

### Team Work! Conquer synergy and make 1+1=3

The collective performance of a team is always the product of two factors: a qualitative and a quantitative one.

There is a big difference between working in groups and work as a team. There are five values that will determine if your team is really a TEAM.

1. Generosity. Generosity means giving the team more than what the team expects from you. Supposed to be generous in the effort and fight well and fulfill my goals to help others if they can not.

2. Humility. Humility means not wanting to always be the star. Sometimes you need to give prominence to others and give a step back to a second term. Let others shine and accept their help will mean eventually that even today I do not have a good day, I will allow others to help me achieve collective goals.

3. Confidence. Confidence in a team is similar to the strength of a table. The more legs it has, the stronger it is. When we talk about confidence, each leg equals every time we do something right and we realize we did it. Some people do well the thing but does not realize this, and so, never comes to have personal confidence. For the team to have confidence it is important to celebrate each success be it large or small. So when a team has confidence, every time it faces a big challenge ahead it will be able to take that first step.

4. Enthusiasm. Enthusiasm is the philosopher's stone for a team. Enthusiasm is the ingredient that makes everyone feel like participating and being generous with others. Enthusiasm is contagious, but the lack of enthusiasm also is! so the maximum number of team members must show enthusiasm and spread it to others.

5. Commitment. Commitment appears when fun is over. Show commitment of continuing to maintain the other four values when things get difficult and easy and leave. Commitment is what really sets the good teams of high performance teams.

When we live the five values, the magic of synergy occurs. When team members are enthusiastic, everyone is inspired to be generous in the effort. Therefore, all give a little bit more than what is expected of them. And when we add that little extra effort, it forms the new piece of the team. So one plus one equals three.

And just some final words for emotion. If you master your emotional world you master everything in your life.

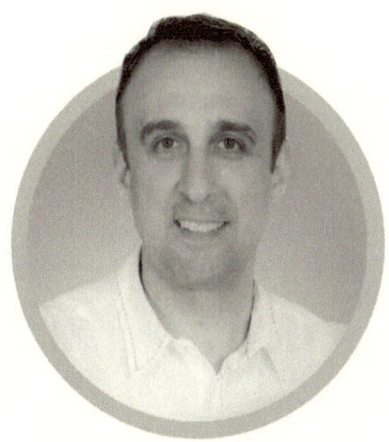

## Xesco Espar

Born in Barcelona (Spain) in 1963. Got a Degree in Sciences of Physical Activity and Sport at the University of Barcelona, Master Degree in Psychology of Learning at UAB and Master Degree in High Performance in Team Sports. Professor at the INEFC Barcelona (Sport University) from 1991 to present

12 years experience coaching young athletes, 10 years of experience in the High Performance at FC Barcelona, achieving 8 Spanish Championships and 4 European Champions League.

Currently he works as an expert in Sports Planning, Sports Coaching, Emotional Control and Motivation (www.xescoespar.net) and conduces transformational seminars on personal emotional control and power (www.firewalkbcn.com)

He delivers keynotes, seminars and workshops in Spanish and English on Leadership, Motivation and Teamwork. He has worked with thousands of coaches, entrepreneurs, managers and executives in Europe and South America.

In the last ten years has inspired hundreds of companies to break the limits of their current performance, generating growth and teamwork in pursuit of their boldest goals.

Author of the best seller "Jugar con el corazón" - in English "Play from your heart" (2010). Currently it is in its 13th edition with 25,000 copies sold.

Websites:

www.xescoespar.net
www.academiadeentrenadores.com
www.firewalkbcn.com

Sign-up for our mailing lists to take part on our community of people who sets for not less than changing the world and get the best motivational training available today.

# 4

## BE IN ONE PEACE – 3 DECADES OF DISTILLED INSIGHTS

- BY DR. JOANNE MESSENGER, TRUE AMBASSADOR FOR HEALING: CHIROPRACTOR AUTHOR (BE IN ONE PEACE, HOW TO BALANCE YOUR HORMONES) RETREATS.

I've always landed on my feet. Life has taken it's series of turns, however I've always ended up in the right place at the right time.

I grew up in a small country town in Western Australia. I was the youngest of seven children and my mother was a nurse. When one of my six brothers became seriously ill it was natural my parents took him to a doctor, then another doctor and even more doctors and hospitals. He was diagnosed with scleroderma and continued to deteriorate. A family friend suggested they take Chris to a chiropractor. This was back in the sixties when chiropractors were almost unheard of in Australia, but they took a leap-of-faith and it paid off. Chris not only didn't die, he became a champion swimmer and prefect at his school.

With six older brothers I was particularly competitive. I had to be, just to try and keep up. By the time I was ten I was third in the state for gymnastics. At age twelve I was doing back-saults on the trampoline, landed on the frame and fractured my pelvis. Within a year my period stopped, I had my appendix removed and began gaining weight. My body was in big trouble. At seventeen I was adjusted by a chiropractor and my menstrual period returned and my health began to restore. I was blessed to go on and in later years bare a healthy child.

In my final year of high school I was going to my appointment with the career guidance counselor to decide my best future vocation. I heard a voice from nowhere say, "chiropractic". I listened. I also took a leap-of-faith, and went to Melbourne to study. My desire to learn everything I could about healing and energy was fed by both destiny (three life incidents had steered me to chiropractic college) and a need to find ongoing ways to continue to heal myself of the consequences of my injuries.

### The Seeds of Profession Were Already Planted

I'm known for my easy conversational style and professional persona. I have a "do-what-works" philosophy. I have an innate knack for seeing what people need to do, to get things right in their body and their life.

If they're in physical pain, I often know what they need to do to sort it out. If they have faulty thoughts, toxic beliefs, or unresolved issues, I can often see the root cause and essential steps they need to follow for resolution.

I've dedicated my life to helping people on all levels, by helping them move forward using step-by-step skills and techniques that are based on practical experience.

The best thing I'm known for is a my track record and ability to identify the root cause of my patient's problems. When people tell me their stories it describes the smoke. I'm really good at finding the fire that's causing the smoke, and helping them resolve that.

I love my patients and they're really grateful for what I do for them. They show their appreciation by referring other like minded people who also want help. Word-of-mouth referrals are the best compliment.

## Work, Passion, Purpose – What Comes First?

I've worked with people from many different backgrounds. I mostly work with people like me. People who are sensitive, who've tried a range of healing methods but still need another key to resolve their issues, so they can heal themselves and follow a fulfilling path of purpose.

### Everyone is born for a reason.

I'm most passionate about helping people do what they're here to do— to make sure they don't die with their music still in them. Everybody has a life purpose, a reason to be on the planet. I enjoy helping people find their purpose independently of pressures from what their family, schoolteacher, or spouse thinks.

My purpose includes helping people fulfill their life-purpose with minimum fear and maximum peace. Many people are challenging old paradigms, breaking down barriers and out-dated rules. My job includes helping them to fulfill their ambitions as easily as possible.

I really like working with people who've had trials, tribulations and issues, and are committed to overcoming them. When people work with me, they usually not only get well and stay well, but also thrive in their careers. As they improve they also pay it forward to their children, family, colleagues, neighbors and so on. Every time I help someone, I know I'm also helping everyone connected to them. The ripples spread.

### Spiritual Alignment, Development and Growth

Personally I'm passionate about anything that helps my own spiritual development, alignment, and growth. This largely means meditation and affirmation. Plus, most mornings I run or walk the beach, soak in the bath with essential oils, and do anything that raises my energy, vibration, or supports my body.

I love talking about energy, life purpose, personal and spiritual growth, healing, alignment and nutrition; how to get the most out of meditation so you can connect with your higher self and higher guidance. Its important to align with your higher self rather than doing what your ego craves.

On weekends or whenever I take time off, you'll often find me at the beach. I live only ten minutes away so access is easy.

I love walking on the sand, drinking spicy chai with my friends or going to a comedy movie. I'll go for anything that makes me laugh. You'll never see me at a horror movie. If I'm paying the money it needs to make me feel good.

### How Did It All Start?

I graduated in 1982 so I've been in practice for 33 years, however my education truly started from birth.

When I finished high school there were only two options for chiropractic courses, Melbourne or the United States. Logistics won and I went to Melbourne to study. I've been on the east coast pretty much ever since.

### Volunteer Inclination

I've always loved and supported activities and projects that help women and children. For instance, I've spoken at Women at Work, and helped organize the Women for Women Forums. We hired the town hall, invited speakers, therapists, stall holders and psychic readers so women could come and gain knowledge they didn't previously have access to, for a budget price.

I really like projects like OXFAM where we donate money if we don't have available  time or skills. We donate money for people to buy chickens, goats and plants, or drill wells for water in countries where there's limited access to essential resources.

In Australia, I really like supporting Homeless Connect. It's a group of people who are really dear to my heart. On a regular basis, they hire the city hall and have hair dressers, caterers, photographers, chiropractors, and massage therapists, donate their time and skills so homeless people can come and have a shower, get a hair cut, a chiropractor adjustment, new clothes and have a free meal and generally feel good about themselves. The photographers take photos of the beneficiaries while they are looking good, so that they can feel good about themselves or use it to apply for a job.

### Accolades and Awards Poured In

Although my mum thinks my qualifications are nothing short of stupendous I work in the true sense of the *wounded healer*. It's the things I've had to face and grow from on my journey to health, love and fulfilment that are my credentials in the real world.

"I've Always Been a High Achiever..."

Early Highlights:

- Third in the state for gymnastics by age 10.
- School captain.
- Honours awards in academic excellence.
- Dux of school.
- Citizenship award.
- Accepted into the Melbourne chiropractic college at only 17yrs and graduated top of the class.

Real Qualifications:

- Bachelor Degree in Applied Science (1982)
- Diploma of National Board of Chiropractic Examiners (USA)
- Excellence Award in Radiology
- Diploma of Sacro-Occipital Technique
- Certified Yoga Teacher (RYTA200)
- Certified in Neuro Linguistic Programming (NLP) as applied to education
- Practitioner and teacher certificates in Chiron Healing
- And studied Aromatherapy; Australian Bush Flower Essences; Essences of the Ancient Civilizations; Pleiadean Light Work and Pranic Healing.

Experience Worth a Mention:

- Published *Be in One Peace*
- Published *How to Balance Your Hormones*
- Hosted my own weekly radio program on Highlands FM.
- Regular guest on the Coffee Break TV program
- Past treasurer of S.O.T.O. A/Asia Ltd,
- Founder and teacher of Blueprint Healing.
- Past Principal of the Australian Energy School of Chiron.
- Past Vice President of the International Association of Chiron Healers Inc.
- Taught the philosophies and techniques of energy and healing

internationally.
- Guest speaker at International Flower Essence Conference.
- Guest speaker for Women at Work.
- Co-founder of Women for Women Australia

## What Drives Me

I have a passion for empowering people to help themselves, align with their life purpose and get results, even if they've never felt good enough, have struggled for years or are scared to death of making changes.

My specialty is presenting new paradigms and detailed information with an easy-to-follow and practical format.

Most people know me as *the voice for health* and *the ambassador for living your purpose.*

## Business Breakthroughs

I've successfully published two books, *Be in One Peace* and *How to Balance Your Hormones,* and have 33 years experience as a chiropractor, healer and international course facilitator. I have an athletic desire for results which led me to develop ground-breaking methods and courses which have helped thousands.

I do one-on-one consultations for energy healing including long-distance healings by phone or Skype.

I've recorded meditation CDs so people can help and empower themselves. I blog, make YouTube videos and facilitate meditation and self healing groups. I've previously taught energy healing to practitioners so they can use it with their own clients.

People generally learn more about me from my evolving website www.drjoannemessenger.com and my YouTube channel and Facebook page (links below).

## Message To The World

You get more of what you think about. Make sure your thoughts, words and actions are taking you closer too, not further away, from what you want. Get started now and keep going. Don't die with your music still in you.

Dr. Joanne "Jo" Messenger has been listed as one of Adyar's Great Australian Authors. She's written Be in One Peace, How to Balance Your Hormones, and has over 30 years experience as a chiropractor, Chiron Healer, course facilitator and public speaker.

When Dr. Jo was twelve, she fractured her pelvis in a trampoline fall. The experience inspired in the young woman a desire to learn everything she could about healing, energy and the divine plan.

Now a health care professional, she shares her lifelong quest for healing, releasing karma and living your life purpose – with less fear and more peace.

Dr. Messenger works with people on all levels, helping them move forward by using step-by-step skills and techniques that are based on practical experience.

She knows what its like to want to feel better, and how frustrating that dream can be to attain. The good news is she's gathered all the best tools and techniques that are essential to help get you back on track.

Hormones are messengers– just like Dr. Jo!

Menopause and andropause are not just physical transitions. They're portals to higher octaves within your divine plan, enabling you to reclaim your ancient gifts and knowledge.

Some people fight it and give up; others delve deep and step up.
Which will you be?

With Dr. Messenger you'll find an affinity with her easy conversational style and professional persona. You'll feel she's talking to you personally, guiding you on an important path that will ultimately lead to both physical healing and fulfilment of your divine plan.

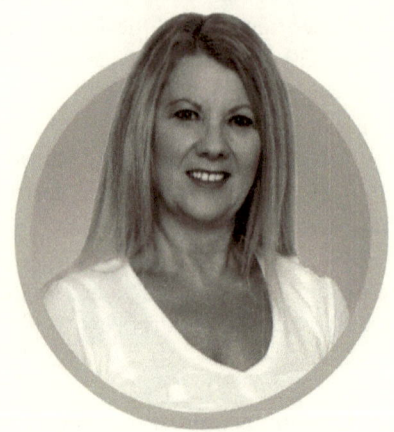

## Joanne Messenger B. App. Sc. (Chiropractic)

802/314-316 Charlestown Rd
Charlestown NSW 2290
Australia
Mobile: 0410 668 070
E-mail: joanne@drjoannemessenger.com
Web: www.drjoannemessenger.com
FB: Dr Joanne Messenger's Be in One Peace

### Personal Information

Nationality: Australian
Place of Birth: Pingelly W.A.

### Summary of Qualifications

| | |
|---|---|
| 1980 | Diplomate, National Board of Chiropractic Examiners U.S.A |
| 1982 | Graduated Phillip Institute of Technology (International College of Chiropractic/ R.M.I.T.) Melbourne. Victoria. Australia. |

|  | B. App. Sc. (Chiropractic) |
|---|---|
| 1982 | Radiology Excellence Award (International College of Chiropractic) |
| 1984 | Diplomate of Sacro-Occipital Technique Awarded by S.O.T.O. A/Asia Ltd. |
| 1983-86 | Primary Instructor for S.O.T.O. A/Asia Ltd. |
| 1991 | Qualified in Neuro-Linguistic Programming as Applied to Education |
| 2000 | BSZ Certificate IV in Assessment and Workplace Training |
| 2008 | RYTA200 Yoga Teacher Training |

## Professional Experience

| 1982 | Western Victorian Chiropractic Centre Warrnambool. Victoria. Australia. Associate Chiropractor |
|---|---|
| 1984-1985 | Treasurer and Board Member Chiropractic Alumni Association P.I.T. (Melbourne)Treasurer S.O.T.O. A/Asia Ltd. |
| 1983-1996 | Private Practice at Western Victorian Chiropractic Centre Warrnambool. Victoria. Australia. |
| 1992 | Speaker at the International Flower Essence Conference Speaker and Master of Ceremonies for Women at Work Speaker and Master of Ceremonies for Women at Work |
| 1993 | Master of Ceremonies for the Chiropractic graduation for the Class of 1993, Royal Melbourne Institute of Technology |
| 1996 | Locum Chiropractor |

| 1992-96 | Speaker and Victorian Convener for Dynamic Growth seminars and the Centenary of Chiropractic, Melbourne and the Gold Coast<br>Chiron Healing Centre, Sydney. Private Practice |
|---------|-------------|
| 1997-2004 | Organizer and presenter of the Be In One Peace courses |
| 2004-2006 | Private Practice Melbourne Vic. |
| 2007 | Associate chiropractor New Lambton (Newcastle) NSW. |
| 2008-2010 | Private Practice Kyneton Vic<br>Yoga Teaching Kyneton Vic |
| 2010-12 | Private Practice Toorak Vic<br>Weekly Health and Well-Being radio show on Highlands fm |
| 2011 | Published Be in One Peace (Balboa/Hay House U.S.A.)<br>Private Practice Gordon, Crows Nest and Charlestown NSW |
| 2014 | Published How to Balance Your Hormones (Balboa/Hay House U.S.A.) |

## Professional Membership

The Australasian Yoga Institute

## Registration/Licensure

AHPRA: 0002150932 (chiropractic)
(N.S.W. Chiropractic registration number: CP 0015501)
(Victoria Chiropractic registration number: 20842)

## References

Dr Mike and Di Dunn
2 Courtney Close Charlestown NSW 2290 Australia
(02) 4943 1887

Dr Gus Gunther
Suite 19, 74 Rawson St

Epping, NSW 2509
(02) 9389 7800

## **Hobbies**

Swimming
Meditation
Writing
Pilates
Yoga
Running
Beach walking

# 5

## NOT ALL WHO WANDER ARE LOST
## THE "RED PORSCHE" DILEMMA

### - BY ABE CHERIAN, PRESIDENT AND CEO OF MULTIPLE STREAM MEDIA.

As the gigantic delivery truck lowered its platform and carefully rolled down this gleaming red, high performance sports car, I wondered to myself if I was dreaming. The 1992 Porsche 911 Turbo, that I had until now only seen in magazines (and my dreams), was suddenly parked out front of my tiny one-bedroom Queens, New York apartment. My stomach turned over as I wondered to myself how this could really be mine. I felt totally undeserving of this extremely expensive gift given to me by someone I had met online only a month prior.

The "gift" was from a female friend from Garland, Texas for whom I was helping develop a website. She had recently taken over her family's cotton trading business and was looking for someone who could help get her onto the web. I offered my help, and thus begun a business relationship with a bit of a personal twist. Through our correspondence, she began to open up to me, letting me in on her deepest personal thoughts. These thoughts expressed the turmoil she was feeling inside, her fear and paranoia, as well as the morality she felt about her own sexuality. Being gay isn't always easy coming from a conservative Texas family, and she was facing conflicting morals as she tried to do what was right for her own personal truth.

Because I had helped her with the website, and receptively opened up to her on a personal level, she decided she wanted to surprise me with an extravagant gift. She let me know ahead of time, yet did not tell me it was the car of my dreams until the day she shipped it. Knowing I was already struggling just to pay rent at the time, I felt immediately that this "gift" was quite a strange token of thanks to say the least.

I wondered how I was going to drive and maintain a Porsche when I was hardly maintaining *myself*. I also asked myself over and over why this woman, who was practically a stranger, would spend this much money on someone she hardly even knew? Self-validation, I imagine, comes in different forms for different people. Although she meant well, I later realized this "gift" was more for her than it was for me. Sending me the Porsche was simply a matter of her taking whatever measures she found appropriate to feel better about herself.

Before coming to this conclusion, I tried to refuse this strange gesture, but she wouldn't take no for an answer. She tried to reassure me by telling me how much I deserved this car and that I should start to learn how to accept the good things in life. This "good thing" however, didn't feel so good at all. This car weighed huge on not only my conscience, but on my dire financial situation at that time.

Its not that driving the car wasn't easy. Driving the car was a blast. Holding onto the car in New York City was another matter entirely. Not only did I have to rent a garage to keep the thing from being stolen, but had to pay an arm and a leg for the insurance. The New York City cops didn't make things any easier, either. I would get pulled over for speeding, even if I was going with the flow of traffic. I guess there's just something about a shiny red Porsche that screams "pull me over."

I decided I had to do something. As good as the car should have made me feel, it was making me feel anything but. I thought about selling the thing, but it didn't sit well at all with my conscience. After some time deliberating on what I should do, I decided to send the car back to the woman who gifted it to me. The moment it was picked up to be taken back to Texas, I physically felt a huge weight being lifted off my shoulders. Although I knew she meant well, I could not be the scapegoat to justify her self-worth.

I believe there are lessons in everything, and this Porsche and everything it represented came as one of the most valuable lessons in my life. Although I hadn't asked for anything from this woman, something in my energy must have told her I needed it. In a sense, I imagine I did, because in the end I realized one of the greatest lessons that helped put me in the place I am today. *Never stand begging for that which you have the power to earn.* I learned this power was within me, and from that day on, my life changed dramatically.

I have since owned several exotic cars, and never once have I felt out of place driving them. There has been no anxiety in enjoying things that I know I have earned, and things have changed so much in my life since then in regard to what I own, including my own self-worth. My life is full, and so much has changed since this experience that happened over twenty years ago. There have been so many circumstances, events, and situations that have propelled me to where I am now. My name is Abe Cherian, and this is my story.

## "A Journey of a Thousand Miles Must Begin with a Single Step." Lao Tzu

Born in 1968 to a middle-class family in India, I credit my parents for doing a fantastic job raising not just me, but my two sisters as well. They did the best they could by trying to demonstrate a well-balanced life so we could go into the world with poise and balance. The values they instilled have stayed deep within me until this day. It is because of them that I hold the cultural, material, and spiritual values I am proud to maintain.

It was early on in life that I realized achieving financial success is as simple as knowing the market's wants and needs. I also found out that working effectively to package, present, and deliver these wants and needs as good as I could was just as important as knowing what was in demand. This I learned from my father, and to this day could not be more thankful for the life he demonstrated.

As an entrepreneur his entire life, I watched my father start businesses that he has taken to great heights. I have also seen him on the verge of bankruptcy and total despair. As I saw him go from selling clothes on the street in his early years to owning one of the most successful retail outlets in the city years later, I realized he accomplished everything he did through hard work and an intensely strong discipline.

After high school, I was unsure of what I wanted to do with my life. I was lost as to what my strengths were, so decided I would travel to help broaden my mind and give myself a deeper sense of what direction I wanted my life to take. What I did know was that I did not want to do as most traditional Indian families do and adopt a "secure" profession.

## Not All Who Wander Are Lost

I decided the best course to "find myself" would be to enroll in courses somewhere in Europe. This, I thought, would give me ample opportunity to travel, allowing me to find exactly what it was I was searching for. With the help of my very supportive parents, I enrolled in a three-year course study for Hotel and Restaurant Management. While taking these courses in Switzerland, I knew that I would never pursue anything that had to do with the hospitality industry. I only knew that I wanted to travel and experience as many other cultures as I could around the world.

For seven years from the ages of 17-25, I was given the opportunity to search for what I was looking for. In this time, I studied, travelled, and worked around Europe and London with several chain hotels. Although fun and exciting, this time was also stormy and often very unstable for me. Through everything I learned, I know I would never trade these experiences for the world. This foundation has led me to where I am today, teaching me countless lessons that I still continue to learn from and apply to the present moment.

It was in 1995 that I migrated from Europe to the United States, with the hope of taking on yet another phase of adventure in my life. These hopes however, were overrun by what I felt was an obligation to my family. With the Indian tradition comes certain expectations, and my parents were no different. There is a huge responsibility toward family, and to prove my loyalty to my parents, I agreed to settle down and prove that I could be a son they were proud of.

It wasn't long before my life drastically changed. I suddenly found myself with a new job and new bills, not to mention a new wife and new family members. I felt I was living a life that was not my own and it wasn't long before the rug was literally pulled out from underneath me. It wasn't even two years later that I was divorced and left with $20,000 in debt. I was left in an extremely toxic environment with my ex-wife's family and did the only thing I could think of. I left.

I did not want to let my parents down, yet I could not return to the hospitality industry that left me feeling empty. I only wanted to get as far away from the depressing life I suddenly found myself in and start something new. Instead, I did what most people in my situation do that can't find a job. I went into sales. Not just any sales, but "door-to-door" sales. My life seemed to go from bad to worse overnight, yet I tried to keep my head up and find some kind of humor in my new situation.

*"A salesman knocks on the door of a home and it's answered by a twelve year-old boy with a cigar in one hand and an empty bottle of scotch in the other. The salesman asks the boy, 'Excuse me, son, but is your mum or dad in?' The boy looks at the salesman as if he's crazy and replies 'Does it fucking look like it?'"*

*"A salesman knocked on my door today. "Who currently provides your internet?" he asked. "My next door neighbor," I replied.*

With my new position as a door-to-door salesman, I seriously ran into several comical incidents just like this pretty much every week. As funny as it seems now, at the time it only felt like one rejection after another. I felt like I was literally learning from the school of hard-knocks. Fifty to eighty knocks a day was doing the best it could to help me figure out how I could make things work another way.

At the time, I was working for an advertising company in Long Island that had carved out a pretty nice niche for themselves in the local marketplace. They offered businesses the opportunity to advertise on local supermarket shopping carts and on the back of cash register receipts. I was the guy responsible for selling this niche to the people who were thought to need it.

This was not, mind you, an easy job. Meeting people who were strangers and trying to break the ice was just the beginning. I had to then try to sell the product, convincing them it was something they needed. A huge benefit for their company, I would tell them. I was met with a lot of rejection, yet still had to keep a positive attitude for the next business I would visit. it is definitely a rare breed that can keep their patience and maintain a great attitude while being met with rejection day after day.

The sales job, however, was not without its advantages. Some of the skills I learned while immersing myself in this crazy position truly gave me what it has taken to build an independent life for myself. One of the strongest lessons I took from this time was the obvious push needed to "think outside the box." This mindset has truly instilled me with the much needed confidence and boldness required to start my own ventures and become the successful businessman I am today.

During this time, I also learned how to ask good questions. One question I remember asking potential clients was how many of their potential clients shopped at the grocery store in their area. I then asked them how much they would like these people lining up to buy their stuff. These questions almost always led business owners to think about the potential in what it was I was trying to sell. When I had gotten their attention this way, I was simply someone that could get more clients to their door.

I also realized that in order to be a successful salesman, I needed to know how to listen. Most salesmen are fast talkers. It seems to be something that is almost expected of them. The reasoning behind this is that people think fast talkers are more persuasive, but I'm not too sure about that. I think that one of the best attributes a sales person can have is the ability to be a good listener. The most basic and powerful way to connect with someone else is to truly listen to what they have to say. The most important thing we can give someone is often just our undivided attention.

Toward the end of my "career" as a salesman, I knew in my heart that I could not spend my life on the streets selling things. Although thrilling to live on the edge and meet new people, I never saw myself doing this for more than a year or two. I knew it was time to move on. Moving on, it would turn out, was one of the best decisions I ever made.

### Moonlighting in the New Frontier

*"The critical ingredient is getting off your butt and doing something. It's as simple as that. A lot of people have ideas, but there are few that decide to do something about them. Not tomorrow. Not next week. But today. The true entrepreneur is a doer, not a dreamer."*
*Nolan Bushnell*

I knew I had to do *something*. When I walked away from my marriage almost twenty years ago, the only things I took with me were my Compaq 200 MHZ Pentium Pro computer, a few essential items of clothing, and my books. Perhaps it was the fact that my computer took up the entire back seat of the cab that made my decisions what they were. Sometimes, I think when you break ties and burn bridges it's a good thing. That way, there is no turning back and nothing left to hold you there.

In 1997, there was a lot of talk about the internet and the possibilities it held for e-commerce. If this buying and selling on the internet was to go mainstream, it meant there was already money to be made online. Researching this possibility, I came across a company that sold a comprehensive e-learning system for teens that offered a $7 commission for each customer that was referred to them. Internet sales at that time was nothing what it is today. I had to learn how to reach people, and reach them quickly if I was to find any success working for this company.

Since I had been active in many AOL forums from the start-up days of the internet, I wanted to see if I could make these sales from people I already knew. I make a couple sales from this forum, but always attributed it to people feeling sorry for me. In these beginning days of the world wide web, people were not as trusting as they are now giving out their credit card information online. This made it extremely difficult to close sales, and doing follow ups with potential clients was literally the only chance I had to convince them that the company I was working for was legitimate.

A lot has changed on the internet since its beginning. Back in these days, spamming was not only considered a justifiable strategy, but was actually encouraged. Collecting lists of email addresses and sending them offers was a go in the minds of most online marketers. For a while I worked hard, reaching hundreds of people by going down these lists and sending individual emails. I suppose it worked good enough at the time; I was able to make a few sales, but realized it was far too much work.

I found some progress in a software program called "Group Mailer", and I was able to literally send hundreds of people information with the click of a button. What a concept! The party didn't last long however, and pretty soon ISP's were catching up and most marketers were forced to stop this practice.

In this time, I realized there were seriously thousands of people online searching for ways they could make money through the internet. This was literally the dawn of the "Gold Rush" period online, and just like the Gold Rush of the 1800's, many people were being scammed and cheated. For the many scam artists and cheats out there, there were still a few legitimate companies that paid their affiliates on time and deeply cared about their online reputation. In the midst of crisis, there is always hope.

**Selling Picks and Shovels**

Back in the day, there were thousands of people who gave up their "normal" lives and moved out west with the dream of making a fortune digging for gold. Everyone knew that just one good find could make them rich beyond their wildest dreams. Not everyone was so lucky, and not very many made the fortunes they were looking for.

A funny thing happened along the way, though. There were some very smart witted people who figured that there was another way to make a lot of money from the gold rush that had nothing to do with digging or panning for gold. Those gold seekers needed the tools necessary to chase their dreams and there had to be someone to supply them. Picks and shovels were a hot commodity in the days of the gold rush, and the people that sold them ended up doing just as good as some of those that struck it rich.

The online marketing business was not much different in its "gold rush" stage. There was a need for finding good tools and resources that would generate leads and customers. Just like those that were selling picks and shovels during the gold rush, there were a few that were succeeding online that knew the right tools to use. The ones who didn't were dropping off like flies.

Along with some others that were full-time online marketers, I saw the light at the end of the tunnel. Among these people were computer programmers, online marketers, and web designers, all of whom saw the potential in selling the tools and resources necessary to help people succeed in online business.

To make my own life easier, I started compiling resources and categorizing them in order so they'd be easier for me to find. This was "pre-Google", and people had to search for hours to find the right tools and resources for their business. I decided to share what I had categorized with others, finding that this was an extremely valuable service for those in the same situation as I.

I took what I found to the next level and created my first online based membership services. SupportPros.com was launched and with it I was able to help thousands of people who needed these services. On this site, I offered a membership based forum where people could pay a small fee to gain access to organized resources all in one area. Within the first month, I had made my investment back and then some. This single idea gave me what I needed to focus on the next step of my life without having to worry about what I would do to make ends meet.

### Being in the Flow

Between 2001 and 2008, I experienced tremendous success both in business and my own personal life. Have you ever found yourself so completely immersed in what you're doing that you lose track of time? This is what I experienced in these seven years, and truly felt I was in flow with the natural rhythms of life. I had found my way, and with my dedicated focus, I found success to follow.

In my business life, I combined my knowledge of online advertising with my knowledge of building SAS (software-as-service) programs, and was able to launch numerous small business platforms online. So successful was what I created that I was able to build an in-house team and rent my own office space.

The team I built was a group of "product centered" professionals, all of whom had a keen eye for customer satisfaction. With the help of this amazing team, we were able to create advertising networks and email list management tools for the internet marketing community. Through this, we were able to help tens of thousands of online marketers and small businesses use these platforms to increase leads and sales for their businesses. Many of these businesses are still going strong to this day, and I can't help but feeling a sense of elation in helping them reach these goals.

At the same time, my personal life was flourishing. I met the woman of my dreams, and between 2000 and 2008 we had four beautiful children. Needless to say, we were on top of the world at this time, which is something I imagine just "happens" when you are in the flow. The experience of this flow in both professional and personal pursuits leads to increased positivity, greater performance, and a commitment to long-term, meaningful goals. Although we all experience this blissed out state at some point in our lives, it wouldn't be fair to mention such success without touching on its challenges.

### Taking the Good with the Bad

*"When we least expect it, life sets us a challenge to test our courage and willingness to change; at such a moment, there is no point in*

*pretending that nothing has happened or in saying that we are not yet ready. The challenge will not wait. Life does not look back. A week is more than enough time for us to decide whether or not to accept our destiny."*
*Paul Coelho*

While everything was shining bright and going as smooth as silk for those seven years, in 2009 I hit a wall. One of the hardest things for an entrepreneur is the sudden absence of creativity due to financial stress and monetary obligation. Unexpected changes in the economy during this time really shook things up, and the flow I had been experiencing seemed to cease completely.

Due to the fact that we were primarily a business-to-business service, the shift in the economy certainly affected us in more ways than one. Many of the small businesses we catered to started heavily cutting down on their advertising budgets. The result? Our revenue began to cut down with it.

This drastic cut in revenue instilled a lot of fear and anxiety in me. All of a sudden my world was coming out from under me, and I had no idea what to do. My team felt it to, and the tension between us grew. It was in the beginning of 2010 that with great humility, I had to let go of everyone that was part of my in-house team and try to move forward alone. With all the hardship entailed, I did learn a valuable lesson through it all. You can't be "winning" all the time.

No matter how optimistic we are as entrepreneurs, there are outside forces that are always going to try and limit what we are capable of. This is true in anything in life, and as an independent businessman, I have truly experienced this more times than I would care to admit. Competition, regulations, and technology changes can all quickly change and adversely affect your business and cash flow right along with them.

The regulations I could handle. I had been in the business long enough to know that these are constantly changing. Technology is another component of my business that is also in a constant state of change, and something that I am used to. However when these components change dramatically at the same time, there is little a business can do to cease sudden falls in revenue. Oftentimes, these drastic changes will phase a business out completely.

To put things a little clearer, let me give you an example. The majority of our revenue came from keeping constant contact with our subscribers using email. From 2012 on, there have been dramatic changes in regulation and technology in how email is delivered. So drastic have these changes been, that the result is communication with clients and customers quickly cut, resulting in loss of revenue. There is no doubt that email is evolving into one of the most profitable commodities for large telecommunication corporations, but for those that are involved in online businesses, the change has been more than a little disruptive.

### Lessons Learned Along the Way

In being an entrepreneur for most of my life, I have found that this profession is not without many lessons that go right along with it. I am constantly learning, and this learning has led me down many different avenues encouraging not just to learn more about business, but more about myself as well.

One thing I have learned is that entrepreneurs are not always in a positive state of mind. Is anyone? While no one can truly predict the future, there are entrepreneurs that like to think they're able to. Limitation is an ugly word for those trying to make it on their own, but something that must be realized if there is to be lasting success. These limitations we all experience remind me of a quote by Jim Rohn, one of my favorite people in the self-improvement field.

*"For a farmer, springtime is his most active time. It's then when he must work hard around the clock, up before the sun and still toiling at the stroke of midnight. He must keep his equipment running at full capacity because he has but a small window of time for the planting of his crop. Eventually, winter comes when there is less for him to do to keep him busy."*

This quote has always resonated with me, because sometimes as growing businesses, we tend to forget that the slower times (winter) will soon fall upon us. When are businesses are young and prospering, we tend to think they will always be busy (spring). It is pertinent to know as entrepreneurs that we must be wise and conservative in all seasons. Our decisions and actions should always be delegated with the fact that slower times could be right around the corner, and we should always be prepared for such.

I have personally learned many lessons when faced with unexpected challenges. It has not always been easy and I have made many mistakes along the way. I have tried to change people who haven't wanted to change, realizing that a person will only change when they are ready. We all have certain priorities, and there are times in our lives when our priorities will be vastly dissimilar.

As an entrepreneur, I was also under the delusion that I must wear multiple hats to run a business. When I first started out, I believed I must do everything by myself. This would be the only way, in my mind, that I would reach the success I was aiming for. Rather than wearing multiple hats, I realized what I truly needed was to multiply my time. The only way to do this was to hire responsible employees that would allow me the time I needed to become a success.

One of the biggest mistakes I believe I made during these hard times, was letting my fear control me. Fear is an energy with one of the lowest vibrational frequencies and is toxic to our entire beings. This mental poison does nothing but contaminate the subconscious mind and destroy our self-confidence. Fear is nothing but an agent to increase all our miseries in abundance.

We will all be faced with challenges. Without them, we would not know what it was to appreciate the good that life does bring. When challenges enter our lives, rather than looking at them with fear, we must find the awareness within that our lives are about to take us on an entirely new path. Perhaps this path is the one that leads to our true calling, and one that gently guides us to our ultimate destiny.

### Success Made to Last

*"Most people think that they are prosperous only when they have plenty of money, but real success means to have all things at your command-the things that are necessary for your entire existence."*

For the past several years, I have been searching. What I am searching for is not the next big advertising platform or to make money from the newest technological ideas. While these have potential to blossom into a multi-national corporation, it is something else that I am looking for. What I am searching for is success that will last a lifetime.

The business I love has become partially self-sustaining in recent years. I refuse to give up. My girlfriend and I work a full-day, everyday, managing what we have. We work with a team of outsourced professionals that we are eternally grateful for. It is through their hard work and determination that we are able to focus our time on new ideas where we can help each other and continue doing what we love.

At this point, I am in it for more than discovering my innate ambition and learning new money making methods. I feel that I must do something every single day that will satisfy the cosmic plan for which we are all sent to the earthly plane. I think the reason that most people are unhappy is because they forget to harmonize their material life with the duties and demands of the greater cosmic plan. This is the plan that demands we satisfy our souls not only by doing that which makes us happy, but by increasing the happiness of those that need it most. Through all of this, I have realized before I may love and help others, I must learn to love and help myself.

## The Value Found in Silence

After the economy collapsed and I was forced to let my team go, I found the practice of daily meditation and self-reflection began to slowly start to transform me from within. Although I have been self-reflective since I was divorced in 1999, I didn't think of this seriously until about four years ago. It was then I began a daily practice of meditation and started to understand that there were numerous realms in my own being that I had never fully explored.

The real lasting success and freedom that we all desire can only be experienced in these inner realms. It is here that we are met with our truth, and discover within what it truly means to be a success. To understand the value of meditation, we must understand the value of silence. In the stillness silence brings, we are able to see things as they are, without the distractions not only from the outer world, but also from within our own minds. It is these distractions that are meant to keep us from finding our own true selves.

It is through the practice of meditation that we are offered the opportunity to find our innate inner nature and the truth of the person we are. Our minds create our reality, and retreating from the distractions of the outside world where we can create any reality we desire is one of the most beneficial things that meditation offers us.

It is only through the silence of our minds that we are able to create what we want in our life. No one is forced to do anything they don't want. We all have choices. It is up to us, and only us to choose what we feel at any given moment, no matter what is going on around us. Remember, you can choose to be happy, sad, angry, or full of joy at anytime you wish.

## The Realization of Self

*"Is there a power that can reveal the hidden roots of riches and uncover treasures of which we have never dreamed? Is there a force that we can call upon to give health, happiness, and peace of mind? I believe that the path of self-realization is the only true and lasting way. There are really not many things in life that are guarantees of true happiness. As all things change and have no permanency in our lives-only 'self' is permanent, and so realizing 'self' is ultimate success."*
*Paramahansa Yogananda*

Searching for the "self" can prove to be far less easy than it may sound. Finding the time to silence the mind and search within is difficult if the basic needs of life aren't met. What are life's basic needs? We tend to think of these only as food and shelter, but our basic needs run much deeper than just these two small pieces of the whole.

Some of our most inherent needs as humans are not only food for the body, but food for the mind and soul as well. Our health can be met with food for the body, mind, and soul but this food must be of the highest nutritional content, well balanced and full of the rich nutrients and vitamins we need to sustain our highest selves. Through this sustainment comes the power to concentrate, which is another basic need if we are ever to be of lasting success.

Having an understanding heart and people we can share this with are also truly some of our most basic needs. Without heart and friends to connect with, our souls wither to a fraction of their true essence. Wisdom in action is another one of our basic needs, for without it we tend to continue to make the mistakes that keep us from living in a successful way.

It is only until we develop our own personal power to get what we need, can we truly get what we want. We must do whatever it takes to satisfy our immediate needs, and transcend the urges that tell us to do otherwise. We may used learned skills, tactics, and other strategies we've picked up along the way to try and gain this personal power, but it never seems to stick around when gained through this manner.

You may think of the material successes you've experienced are a tell-tale sign of the personal power you possess. Yes, material success can be a stepping stone to other successes in our lives, but true personal power can only come from within. It is only through conquering self that we can truly have it all.

## Living with Grace

I believe in life, we should realize when we "get lucky." As much as we would like to think that the successes in our lives are because of our great minds and brilliant moves, we may be sadly mistaken. Thinking back upon my own life, I did not strategically plan anything at all. What I did do, however, was become receptive to the universal law of cause and effect and allowed grace to enter into my life. There is no true progress that can be made without truly being conscious of and living with grace.

In grace, we find a certain compassion in living with the world. To live gracefully, we conduct our lives in a tactful manner, respectful of both the people and circumstances that make up our lives. Grace can mean many things to many different people, and is often a difficult concept for many to understand. In my own personal life, I have found the that understanding the deeper meaning of grace, at the very least, makes us more resilient to the challenges life undoubtedly brings.

To me, grace seems to take the form of accidental occurrences that we may not always recognize as blessings. Grace may manifest itself in the form of suffering due to loss, a profound spiritual experience, or perhaps as a feeling of great peace that descends over your being. This can be thought of as spontaneous grace, and we may attribute it to a force or entity outside ourselves. While this is often the case, there is also a point where we reach state of conscious grace, one that is brought upon only through experience, and something we should pride ourselves with sharing with the world around us.

## A New Social Media Revolution SpiritualityWeb.com

Finding a vocation that is in line with our personal philosophy is difficult for many of us to do. As life progresses on, we tend to move further and further away from the dreams of our childhood and our core desires. This, however, can be changed. By using the power of our thoughts and our dynamic will, we can turn things around realize that we truly have the power within to live our life's purpose.

This, I believe, is easier to do when we have others to share and support our dreams and desires. For well over a year I have strategically been planning on how to connect people who wish to live their truth and turn their dreams into reality. I now sit poised, ready to start the next phase of my professional life, helping people do just this.

SpiritualityWeb is a social media platform that is much like Facebook and other social sites. The difference, however, is that it is a place solely for likeminded people who are searching for truth on their spiritual journey. SpiritualityWeb is a place where one can connect, share, and inspire without the distraction of negative influences. I graciously welcome you to visit www.SpiritualityWeb.com and help us all unite.

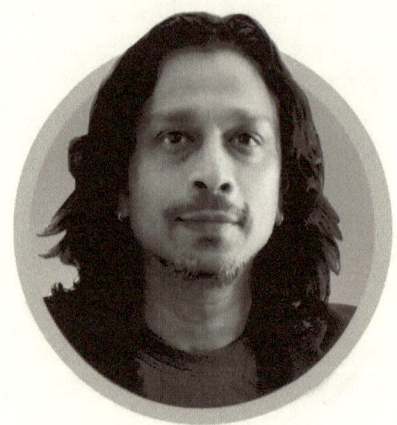

## Abe Cherian

Abe Cherian is the President and CEO of Multiple Stream Media.

Ad Network Platform: http://AdClickMedia.com
Email List Platform: http://liststream.net
More About Abe: http://en.wikipedia.org/wiki/Abe_Cherian

What's New?

Abe is currently focusing on developing a social media platform for non-denominational spiritually oriented people worldwide. SpiritualityWeb.com is a social media platform, much like Facebook or any other Social sites - but it is a place for likeminded people who are searching for their spiritual journey. It is a place where you can Connect, Share, and Inspire others without getting distracted by negative influences.

You are welcome to visit SpiritualityWeb.com and help us unite. http://spiritualityweb.com

# 6

## THE KEY TO MY SUCCESS?

- BY GREG HAGUE, 5-STAR AMAZON REVIEWED AUTHOR, DYNAMIC SPEAKER AND NICHE BUSINESS ENTREPRENEUR.

Upon receiving the invite to write a chapter for this book I thought, "Wait a minute, how **DID** I do it?" That implies I'm done. Not even close.

Barring a medical miracle, I am in the second half of my physical life, but not my accomplishment life. While I am financially fortunate, I don't aspire to retire, never have. In fact, I probably work harder now than I did when I "needed to."

### FAMILY & FRIENDS

Clearly, the #1 factor in my success has been the support and

77

encouragement of my family and friends. My wife, Roseann, has been amazing. I can't imagine any woman who believes in a man more than she believes in me. I can't imagine any wife who could work harder or more unselfishly to help her husband.

My sons, Brian, Corey, Casey, and nephew Jason, have also been there for me at every turn. When they were just kids they understood and didn't make me feel badly when sacrificing vacations because I felt I had to stay back and work. They've pitched in over the years to help in multiple ways, never expecting or asking for anything in return. I'm one lucky dad.

And my friends are the best a man could have. Their willingness to help me, their unwavering confidence in me, and their boundless fountain of support and savvy is more than any human being has a right to expect. Thank you.

## CHUBBY RULES

In addition to family and friends, a key factor to my success has been the advice of some very smart people. It started with my dad (his nickname was Chubby).

A truly fascinating thing about Chubby was that he had to "get smart" because he started life behind the eight ball. Chubby's father died when he was just three. He lived alone with a working-poor mom, attending a rough, lower tier high school.

After training fighter pilots in WWII, he married my mom and started selling real estate with no experience, no one to mentor him, no connections and no open doors. Yet Chubby made millions, built a 300-person firm, bought a bank, flew his own private plane and was considered one of the smartest men in town.

Chubby was a standout example of the difference between being educated and being smart. This meant having a set of strategies that helped him make better decisions, fewer mistakes and know what to do when others were lost in the dark. After he died, I affectionately and respectfully named his strategies "Chubby Rules."

While I didn't realize it at the time, Chubby gave me an imaginary suitcase. Day by day, week-by-week, he filled it with his Chubby Rules, business and life smarts that have helped me hugely virtually every single day of my life.

For over 45 years, I've carried my Chubby Rules suitcase everywhere I go. Not a day goes by that I don't pull out more than one rule and apply it to help me know what to do.

So what exactly is a Chubby Rule? Dad was big on aphorisms (a fancy word for a short phrase that expresses a true or wise idea). But his aphorisms were bigger than that definition suggests. Each Chubby Rule is a "clarity guide", a one-sentence rule I can apply to know precisely what to say and do when others may not.

Over the years, my Chubby Rules suitcase has expanded. While it started with Dad's lessons, I've added a treasure trove of wisdom from my own experiences and from some very smart people I am fortunate to know.

In honor of my dad, and in the hope that they might help you as much as they've helped me, I am sharing two of my favorites. They clarify my way and continue to guide me every day:

## RUSH WITH GOOD NEWS, DRAG YOUR FEET WITH BAD

Most of the world operates in reverse. Read the newspapers. As soon as something bad happens, telephones light up and media trumpets the news. People become glued to the TV screen and seem addicted to spreading the bad news nonstop.

On the other hand, when something good happens, there doesn't seem to be such a rush. The attitude is, "Oh, that's nice, let's move on."

Chubby taught me to do just the opposite. He said to rush with good news the second I hear it (before it could turn to bad). On the other hand, he advised to delay sharing bad news as long as I could, and to not share it at all unless it was absolutely necessary.

Dad's point was that there is no point in being a harbinger of lousy news, stuff you can't do anything about. Why share doom and destruction with people who have no ability to improve the situation? Our time on earth is so limited and precious, it's crazy to waste a minute consumed with negative, depressing or unfortunate news.

Dad also pointed out that sometimes, if you give it time, bad news can turn good, such as when people change their mind and say yes or after they originally said no. Have you ever gone away on vacation and upon returning learned about problems you would have been saddled with, but had already been solved?

Dad also mentioned that with some kinds of bad news, we must tell those who are effected and need or deserve to know. But, he advised to first think about and work on the issue, because I may be able to make it better before I have to tell anyone the news.

For example, while in college and law school I sold real estate part-time to make extra money. Occasionally, I received calls from lenders saying that they had turned down my buyer for a loan. (That was back in the days when lenders weren't obligated to notify the customer before their real estate agent.)

I noticed that most agents would immediately call their buyer with the bad news. Not me. I remembered the Chubby Rule and always tried to first remedy the problem with that lender or have the buyer's application sent to a new lender with more liberal standards.

I might even contact a motivated seller who wouldn't want to lose the sale to see if they would finance all or part of the loan. The point is not to share bad news until you try to solve or alleviate the problem.

In a nutshell:

Don't waste time reading, watching or listening to negative news unless it directly affects you (or a friend or a client) - or unless you think you can do something about it.

Don't share mean, harmful and negative things that go on in the world, stuff you can do nothing about.

If you receive bad news that affects someone you know, first try to solve the problem, or at least think about how to share the news in the most positive way.

Rushing with good news and delaying bad news has been one of my most  powerful Chubby Rules. It's a strategy that sets me apart and keeps me in a positive mood. It is also a time saver, productivity enhancer and quite frankly, it projects me in the way I want to be seen.

## KNOW WHEN TIME IS ON YOUR SIDE AND WHEN IT'S

## NOT

Some people seem to consistently make better decisions than others. I have learned that this is often not because of some innate ability to choose the best course of action. Instead, it's a result of their sensitivity to whether time is working for or against them. Being constantly cognizant of the influence of time on decisions is a remarkable tool for making better choices and fewer mistakes.

I still vividly remember my first lesson from Chubby on the importance of evaluating the time factor. I had just started selling real estate at Dad's real estate firm in Cincinnati, Ohio. I was newly licensed at 18 years old and on summer break from Miami University, 40 miles up the road.

I had been assigned my first "floor time." That meant I was given a three- hour shift sitting at a special desk by the receptionist's station near the front door. The arrangement for sales agent covering floor time was that if any buyers or sellers called or walked in, they were the floor time agent's to pounce on.

The golden time periods for floor time were weekends, when more people were buying homes. My first slot was a coveted Saturday morning and I was really excited.

Sure enough, the phone rang within minutes after I sat down. It was a nice elderly gentleman. He wanted to interview several agents from different companies and then choose one to list his home. This was awesome, just what I had hoped for. Good listings are the name of the game in real estate sales.

I made an appointment the following evening to meet with him and convince him that my dad's company could do the best job of selling his home. Dad had trained me well. (I figured being the boss's son wouldn't hurt either.)

I couldn't wait to call Dad and tell him that I had made my first appointment. That call didn't go as I had contemplated.

ME:        "Dad, I made a listing appointment during my very first floor time. It's tomorrow night."

Chubby:        "Why tomorrow night? Did you ask if you could go over this afternoon?"

ME:        "No."

Chubby:     "Greg, there is a 50% chance that appointment will cancel.
Some other agent will get in there before you and talk the seller into
listing with him and cancelling with you. From the moment you receive a
call like that time is working against you."

ME:        "What should I do?"

Chubby:     "Greg, you're smarter than that. Pick up the phone and try
to convince that seller to meet you tonight."

Dad's lesson on always thinking whether time was working for or
against me has been a huge factor in helping me make better decisions.
Hiring. Employee bonuses. Buying. Selling. Setting meetings. Whether I
should initiate a call or wait for the person to call me. When the phone
rings, should I take the call or let it go to voice mail?

Consider:

You are buying a car.  Is time on your side?

There is invariably a multitude of car buying choices.  Cars decline in
value as newer models with new features are introduced. Also, once you
buy your options end. The seller can invest and make money on your
money while you are stuck with a depreciating asset.

So is time working for or against you? For you, to be sure.

But there is an exception. What if the car you want is an antique or a
one-of-a-kind? In that case, time is not on your side. If it sells to someone
else, you're out of luck … possibly forever.

Another good example is real estate. People who list their homes for
sale generally have no idea how time hurts them. Sellers rarely realize their
home begins declining in value the moment it's placed on the market. Time
is their worst enemy. Why?

After price, the first thing buyers ask is DOM (how many days the home
has been on the market). Buyers never offer as much for a home that's
lingered on the market a long time.

It makes sense. When a home has been on the market for months, prospective buyers figure other buyers have rejected it because of the price, or possibly because "something" is wrong.

It's a real shame. I've seen homes that were fairly priced end up selling at a lower than fair price because of the time factor. It happens quite often. I've observed hundreds of homes over the years that weren't marketed aggressively by the listing agent, didn't get exposed to many or any buyers, and then ended up selling for less than real value.

Evaluating the impact of time with every decision has been a huge positive for me. Selling or buying are only two of the many examples of how time has influenced my decisions.

Thinking about whether time is on my side or not is one of the most significant Chubby Rules in my suitcase. I consider it every day. Give it a try. I think you'll be surprised at the power of this simple concept.

## **CONCLUSION**

If I can ever help you in any way, think of me as one of your "911s". "Being there" for people in need is one of my key priorities. I believe our meaning on earth is not determined by the money we earn or the mountains we climb, but rather the people we impact in positive ways.

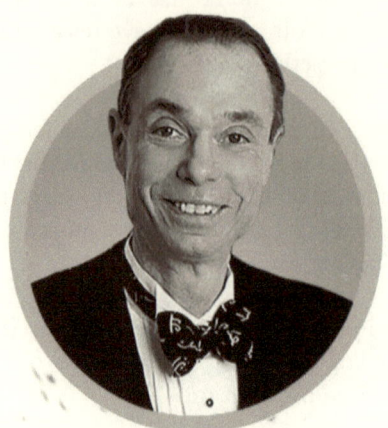

## Greg Hague

Greg Hague is an Avvo rated "Superb" attorney, national real estate authority, 5-star Amazon reviewed author, dynamic speaker and niche business entrepreneur.

Greg received the #1 score when he took the Arizona bar exam, was voted "Law Professor of the Year" by Arizona Summit Law School, was honored as one of Arizona's Top 50 Pro Bono Attorneys and is a founding partner of a law firm dedicated to the needs of entrepreneurs.

Greg was lauded by Real Estate Today magazine as one of America's leading real estate visionaries, having founded several successful real estate firms based on creative business models, including an international referral service, the #1 ranked luxury home brokerage in Arizona and a 122-office national real estate franchise he built starting with three agents in one office. Greg has also been involved in founding a string of successful non-real estate businesses, including Harvey Mackay University, SmartsMatter, Savvy Dad, HKM Law, RapidFire Books and Flexground, a 2014 Inc. 500 Fastest Growing Company.

Greg has served as a business commentator for NPR and expert real estate contributor to The Wall Street Journal. He has appeared in over 100 television and radio shows across the country, was featured in Kiplinger's book, Buying and Selling a Home and in Carolyn Janik's book, Selling Your Home in the 90s.

Greg has been nominated Entrepreneur of the Year, Educator of the

Year, served as a Dale Carnegie instructor and authored the popular book, How Fathers Change Lives - 52 Stories of Remarkable Dads.

Greg has been a keynote speaker at over 450 real estate, corporate and entrepreneurial events including meetings by American Express, Shaklee Products, RE/Max and Century 21. He currently writes and speaks on law, real estate and a concept he developed called "Smartsmanship." Greg is a health advocate, nutrition nut, instrument-rated pilot and motorcycle adventurer, having explored Canada, Europe, Africa and landed his plane on remote Mexican beaches.

Greg is currently a newspaper columnist, law, real estate and business success speaker, partner in Flexground, a 2014 INC 500 company, founder of RapidFire Books, senior partner at HKM Law, and Chief Executive Officer of Harvey Mackay University.

# 7

## MULTIPLE SCLEROSIS, SADIE HAWKINS AND A REDHEADED NERD'S JOURNEY TO BECOMING A RENOWNED TRANSFORMATIONAL LEADER
- BY STEPHANIE MULAC, AUTHOR, SPEAKER, INTUITIVE LIFE COACH.

No childhood story starts out well when you are an awkward redhead with freckles in a private, upper class Catholic school with the church paying your tuition because you are the token charity case. Add to that mix hitting puberty at nine years old and developing faster than half the teenagers in the school; being a nerdy, straight A student (complete with glasses) and for the proverbial icing on the cake, top it all off with the 1960's stigma that goes along with a mother who is divorced.

**Welcome to my childhood.**

It was with all of these "assets" that I began shaping my destiny in a tiny town in southwestern Pennsylvania and where so many lessons would ultimately unfold that would sculpt the person I was meant to be and lay the foundation for the path my life would ultimately take.

My earliest memories of life as a student involved a lot of teasing, ridicule, name calling and even getting beat up on a fairly frequent basis. I recall one time in particular on the playground being surrounded by a group of girls from the upper grades who were pushing and shoving me, pulling my hair and before all was said and done I ended up being thrown down a set of cement stairs leading back into the cafeteria.

Where the nuns were or how this could have been done without anyone intervening is really a mystery to me – all I know is that it was likely how I developed the notion that you can't always rely on someone to be there to pick you up, so fending for yourself in this world was a good skill to develop early on. Of course, at that age, it wasn't quite framed that way, but in retrospect, I think we can all see how easily those types of conclusions can be drawn as a result of childhood experiences. Nevertheless, incidents like this reinforced a survival instinct that got me through many things during my tumultuous school years.

There was another incident I like to share that illustrates how we often have so many negative patterns and beliefs about wealth and abundance injected into our psyche at a young age. It was the middle school rite of passage known as the "Sadie Hawkins" Dance, wherein the girls invite the boys and of course I knew just who I wanted to invite – the other class "brain" who I had a huge crush on. Imagine my elation when he said yes!

The night had all the trappings of puppy love come true - complete with my mom and I getting a special dress at the thrift store, working on styling my hair just right and applying an ever so light dusting of makeup. I left the house feeling like a princess with so much excitement for the night ahead.

My mom pulled up in front of this mansion in our town's most exclusive neighborhood to pick up my date, and I was truly oblivious how out of place we were in those surroundings. In fact, I thought nothing of it. There we were showing up in our old red and black Pinto, which to me was every bit as elegant as a horse drawn carriage and fit to transport me, and my knight in shining armor to the dance. Little did I know that I was about to learn a harsh lesson in class prejudice. In fact, unbeknownst to me, I was the lead character in the middle of my very own Cinderella story.

I beamed as I got out of the car, floating on cloud nine as I headed to the front door and rang the ornate doorbell with excited anticipation. As the door cracked open, a well dressed gentleman began to greet me, but was interrupted from further back inside the house when I heard a woman's voice sharply say, "I don't want that trash in my house, make her wait out on the landing!"

Yes, that was the first time in my life (that I was aware of) that I came face to face with the reality that in some people's eyes we are not all created equal - despite what our daily Catholic studies were teaching my friend and me. I'm not entirely sure what emotions I was feeling right at that moment, the blur of it all would seem to meld heartbreak with rejection, wounded pride and hypocrisy. All I specifically remember was trying to hold back tears, smiling from the porch and looking back over my shoulder at my mother still proudly sitting in our car. I do remember distinctly thinking that she didn't need to hear about what just happened and have her night ruined too, so telling her what I'd just heard would wait until another day.

In that split second on the doorstep, my hopes were dashed that the night ahead would be the start of something more than just a one-time outing. I remember having the time of my life at the dance that night – my date had apparently not been tainted by his mother's prejudice (or maybe he just didn't care), but in any event he treated me like royalty that night and it was truly one of my happiest social memories from childhood - despite knowing in the back of my head that the proverbial clock would strike midnight and I would go back to reality the next day.

And as a rather amusing footnote to this story, I will digress a moment here and share that it wasn't until well over 30 years after graduating that I ever ran across my friend again – and this time it was a picture of he and his 'husband' on Facebook that came up on a mutual friends timeline. I often marvel at the irony that this mom didn't think I was good enough for her son due to my financial stature and yet my guess is that her homophobic tendencies were far greater than her prejudice against poverty. Sometimes I just smile at the sense of humor that the Universe has.

Suffice it to say, my daily life and experiences growing up continued to proceed along a pretty consistent pattern that illustrated how cruel kids can be to one another and how important it is to take what life presents and leverage the experience into something that is beneficial.

The concept of finding the positive in every adversity is probably the most powerful teaching that my mother ever did and it came from within her heart, as she had no formal training in any of the powerful personal growth practices we are all so familiar with today. She always used to just say that every cloud has a silver lining and that I should be thankful to the people who were hurting me because in the end it would only serve to make me stronger. And she was 100% right!

Together, we were the perfect mother daughter duo- facing life head on no matter what the challenge or struggle - and what she instilled in me will forever be with me. It also represents a huge part of what I teach my own daughters as well each and every day.

Until society started harshly pointing out otherwise, I thought my mom and I lived an abundant and luxurious life – little did I know how close we were to poverty level as measured by conventional means. To the contrary, we were indeed rich beyond measure and the values she instilled in me were priceless.

I truly have no idea to this day how my mother made ends meet and how she was able to provide so many things for me. From holiday traditions, to her cooking and baking skills and extending to clothing, necessities and even little extravagances sprinkled in, she must have been a master at budgeting and making a dollar stretch.

For most of my life she was a secretary and I am not sure in any given year that she made over $15,000 to $20,000 a year from a hard earned paycheck. All I ever really knew was that she was highly regarded in the law firm she worked for and was even the first typist who got sent to school to learn how to use a word processor – seen as the most technically advanced office tool of its time. This was such a huge honor that the local paper even wrote an article about her being chosen to learn this new technology and how much it would help the town.

She was well loved by her co-workers and from the outside looking in, it would seem that she had job security for life from an employer who would value the contribution she made to keeping his office, employees and clients happy.

And so life proceeded, she worked many long hours, put in over time and did her utmost to see to it that I had a good education and thus be able to get into a good college and make a better life for myself. In those days, that was the blue collar American dream and she was seeing to it that the script was being written just like it was described in the text books.

That was until life threw my me and my mom another curveball that would forever change my view of the status quo and encourage me to begin writing an "entrepreneurial" script far different than the 9-5 book that all of our parents of that generation read.

I remember in my senior year of high school that my mother started having unusual symptoms like her lip and cheek on one side of her face would get numb or as she described it, her leg would tingle like it fell asleep - but it wouldn't go away for days at a time. She started becoming unsteady on her feet and joked when we went shopping that people would probably look at her and think she was drunk.

This actually went on for a while and her doctor suspected he knew what was going on but an MRI test was the only definitive way to get a diagnosis and her insurance wouldn't pay for the test because it hadn't yet received FDA approval and she couldn't afford to pay for it on her own. So we waited and wondered as her symptoms got worse and as soon as insurance would cover the test, our worst fears were realized.
My mother was diagnosed with MS (Multiple Sclerosis).

I was in college at the time, continuing to live out that American dream we all bought into, and my best buddy - the woman I was supposed to share life with as a young adult and beyond was becoming more crippled by the day – dashing many of the hopes, dreams and plans we once shared together.

What neither of us was prepared for, however, was what was about to happen to her at work. She went from the beloved employee to being treated like a leper with a contagious disease. People's misinformation about MS combined with a boss who only had his eye on the bottom line started a chain of events that were unconscionable.

In spite of the fact that she was perfectly competent to continue working for many years to come, her job was suddenly and mysterious terminated not long after news of her diagnosis came to light. The bottom line was that the law firm didn't want the baggage of someone with an illness and after years and years of dedication and service she was no longer of any value when viewed as "damaged merchandise."

Discrimination, injustice, sheer ignorance? Yes, it had all of those trappings, but to a small hometown girl with no business savvy, it was not even a consideration for her to initiate a court battle against the biggest law firm in town. And to mitigate their damages, they even made a huge ordeal about pulling strings with city counsel to get a handicapped street sign put up so she could park her car closer to her front door on the street where she lived.

So while tradition in those days was being given a gold watch at retirement, my mother got a handicapped sign along with her termination paperwork – indeed putting a new spin on the notion of being kicked to the curb.

Suddenly, the woman who soothed many tears from her little girl who came running home from school with questions of *"why don't they like me,"* and *"why can't I be like everyone else,"* had come full circle. And the strength that she instilled in me all those early years was the strength I drew upon many, many times through the years that followed as I watched this insidious disease take over every aspect of her life and ultimately become the root of the complications she would die from.

During this time though, there was something else transpiring beneath the surface that is directly responsible for who I am and where my passion lies to this very day.

You see, MS is not a death sentence. There are plenty of people who go onto live fulfilling, productive lives even with this disease. But what I witnessed in my own mother's reaction to it all spoke more to the mindset than the body.

Simply put... she mentally gave up.

My mother, the woman who infused me with immeasurable strength to persevere despite all odds... gave up. In fact, she intimated to me one time shortly after her diagnosis that she devoted her entire life to raising me and her "job was now done." She felt like she did her part, and with the diagnosis of this disease it meant that her time on earth was finished and there was no convincing her otherwise. Truly, when she made up her mind and that was her reality, she might have well signed her own death sentence right at that point.

It was at this juncture in my life that I realized how critically important mindset is in our lives and the role it plays. And this realization became more than simply a passing notion - it became my passion to study everything I could about the role the brain plays in our life, success and in manifesting our goals.

In addition, the hard core reality that I witnessed from my mother's employer when she got sick also gave rise to my entrepreneurial spirit and the promise I made to myself that my success in life would never rest in someone else's hands at the mercy of a 9 to 5 job!

Lastly, the final take away here as it relates to my childhood is the importance of taking seemingly negative experiences and turning them into strength and character building experiences, giving us the physical and emotional tools necessary to succeed beyond measure.

Had it not been for the strong love, support and emotional guidance I got from my mother, my grade school and high school experiences would have left me with self esteem lower than low and a belief system surrounding wealth and abundance that was extremely tainted. But instead, I had the well-grounded teaching of a loving and devoted mother who taught me in her own rudimentary way how to overcome all those experiences and leverage them into positive life skills that are solidly with me to this very day.

In reality, I don't see my life experiences as being all that unique – in many ways, most of my clients and friends have similar stories to greater or lesser degrees. What I do see as a separator though is the lack of a support system similar to what I had in my mother. Few people that I've encountered in this world were as fortunate as I was to have someone there to inject balance and perspective into so many life lessons.

As a result, as adults many people reach a point in their life that they need to isolate and dissolve the limiting beliefs and negative patterns that were instilled in them along their life's journey. And this is where my passion for helping others break through the barriers to their own success comes into play. It is my calling and my life's work and where I derive my greatest pleasure in helping others eliminate the dream barriers in their life and leverage their experience in order to sculpt their ideal life.

You see, when we come into this world, we are issued a birth certificate and after our final breath our life is sealed with a death certificate. Truly though, it is the time in between these two pieces of paper that validates who we are and the legacy we will leave. It is in fact our "Life Certificate," and we are writing it each and every day.

It's been a pleasure sharing a part of my own Life Certificate with you and as a token of my appreciation for your valuable time you have spent with me reading my story, I would like to give you a free gift – a short inspirational video that I hope will motivate you to go forth and continue to write your story. Click here to watch it: http://yourlifecertificate.com and please share it with anyone you know who will resonate with the message as well.

In addition, one of my most powerful tools to effect lasting change and to uplift me as I journey my own path in life is the use of brainwave entrainment. Having seen the ill effects that mindset played in my own mother's life, my studies around BWE stemmed from these early discoveries. In fact, I am so passionate about the benefits, that I enlisted the assistance of a great friend to co-co-create http://QuantumMindLibrary.com and I would like to invite you to experience your choice of 477+ audios 100% free with my compliments. No matter what you are pursuing to assist you in your own personal development goals, this is a perfect compliment and it is my pleasure to introduce it to you as well.

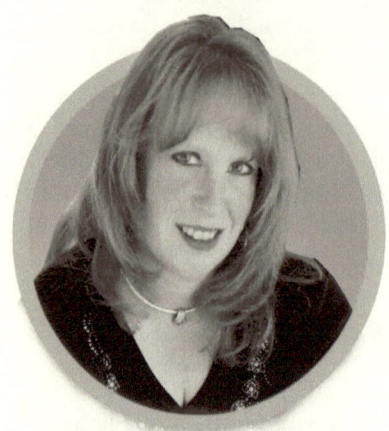

## Stephanie Mulac

Author, speaker, and Intuitive Life Coach, Stephanie Mulac has been a facilitator for 1000s of people worldwide in guiding them to manifest the life of their dreams and lead an extraordinary existence!

As a renowned transformational advisor, Stephanie is best known for rapidly identifying and eliminating the destructive patterns and beliefs holding so many deserving individuals hostage – prohibiting them from unlocking their infinite potential. Her guided, intuitive approach assists enlightened individuals to tap their inner strength and leverage it to bring about accelerated and lasting transformation in all areas of their life.

Founder of the Infinite Evolution Center (IEC), Stephanie embodies the IEC philosophy that *"Prosperity Is Multidimensional."* Her proven methods for developing an equitable balance between mind, body and spirit while pursuing financial abundance utilizes her renowned Milestone Mapping technique – a process by which individuals routinely experience proportionately high success rates when other methods of manifesting have previously proven elusive.

For the past 20 years, Stephanie has been recognized worldwide as a leading expert in the personal growth, marketing and technology space. And for 8 years, she had the distinction of founding and hosting Self Improvement Gifts – an online event responsible for annually assembling over 900 personal growth experts that came together each January for the single largest self-improvement gathering of its kind in the industry.

She is also creator of the acclaimed short movie – Your Life Certificate

– and invites you to watch, enjoy and share it here: http://www.YourLifeCertificate.com

**Personal:**

A huge proponent of leading by example, Stephanie and her family have embraced their own financially free lifestyle as she's traveled full-time by motorhome across the U.S. since 2008, with her then "pint sized" daughters Marina and Morgan – both successful online entrepreneurs, home schoolers and mini-manifestors in their own right.

Maintaining focus, balance, gratitude and a perpetual flow of positive energy is the cornerstone of Stephanie's mindset, and as a tribute to her authenticity, teaching these principles goes far beyond her immediate family – encompassing all with whom she comes in contact.

She routinely and effortlessly manifests her deepest desires, teaches her daughters how to do so as well, and her passion is to teach you to do the same!

Please enjoy this free gift at http://QuantumMindLibrary.com where you will find the most advanced brainwave technology online today with over 477+ MP3 audios available for you to enjoy. There's no limit to how good you can feel and what you can achieve with these sessions and it's Stephanie's heartfelt passion to share them with you as well.

Connect with Stephanie at:
http://StephanieMulac.com
http://facebook.com/stephanieleighmulac
Blog:http://stephaniemulac.com/blog
Email: mulacsites@gmail.com

# 8

## FROM BEGGING TO CHOICE

- BY AXEL MEIERHOEFER , EXPERT IN LEADERSHIP &
BUSINESS DEVELOPMENT HELPING ORGANIZATIONS &
PEOPLE SUCCEED.

My professional career started in the military. I served 22 years in the Air Force, flying fighter jets and serving in more and more leadership and project-related roles. When I retired as a staff officer, the challenge was to become successful in private industry. By my own measure I succeeded, having an executive position in a small software company that developed and offered IT-solutions to diverse industries.

10 years ago I felt a need to prove to myself that I can use my own ideas and ideals to create a successful company. That's when Axel Meierhoefer Consulting LLC, now better known as AMC LLC, was founded. The goal was to offer

coaching/mentoring/speaking as one leg of a three legged stool, program and project management as the second leg, and employee development as the third.

Based on the experience and wisdom of the last 10 years, I have learned a few lessons that I believe will help others on their path to success. I have turned these lessons into 7 principles. Interestingly some of these principles were already in place from the start of AMC LLC and other grew into important cornerstones on the way to how we operate these days.

The one thing I can tell anybody reading this chapter is:
**"There is reason to be hopeful, even if things might not look like it initially".**

When I started I established

**Principle #1: The Core Mindset must be right – serving is everything!**

The AMC LLC motto is: "Helping others help themselves become successful!"

– yes, it is a nice slogan. More importantly it is really a mindset and does have no aspect of 'making money' attached. You might ask yourself how a business can function and become successful with that mindset? The answer is:

**<u>Your focus gets influenced.</u>**

I suggest you always look for the point where you can apply your helping hand, your ideas, your views, your experience, and the things you already know, to provide help. This mindset and the associated actions lead to appreciation. Not always will those receiving your help be able to repay you with money – right away or ever. What they can do is to repay you with their kindness, with any contact they might have that could be helpful to you. They will keep an eye out for your needs and make you aware of opportunities – if for no other reason than to make themselves feel good through giving back some of what they received from you.

I am the first person to admit that keeping this mindset is harder than it sounds. I am grateful to my mentor, David Mark Corbin, for helping me when I was in a dark place beginning to wonder if I will be able to fulfill my dream of a successful company. At the bottom of the recent recession I had

gotten my mind convinced that I am a small dirty beggar who is hoping to get a few crumbs to allow my company to survive and feed my family. I had decided that all the things I had learned and what I had to offer, including a PhD in leadership and organizational change, were obviously not of interest – if they were my client list would be full of great project
s.

Turns out the vibe you put into the universe is the vibe that comes back to you. When David helped me to change my mind-set back to focusing on what I have to offer and portraying it in a desirable way,  business changed within a few months.

When you ask yourself how to transition from Beggar to Choice

**Principle # 2 comes into play: Relationships come before Contracts!**

You might ask yourself what David did to get my mindset straight? – Basically he asked me who I am spending most of my time and energy on and with. This references a book written by a friend of mine, Greg Reid, titled "Three Feet from Gold". My deepest learning from it was – with the help from David:

You, as I do regularly now, have to ask yourself who the 5 people are who you spend a significant amount, if not all your time, with. Are they helping you, motivating you, inspiring you, making you believe and feel energized every day to strive toward the kind of success they already achieved?

If you can't say – from the bottom of your heart and your gut – that these 5 people are your shining beacons guiding you forward, you are hanging out with the wrong people.

Realizing that is easy – and maybe some of your 5 are already in the right category. Making changes to have 5 or more folks that can help you become successful, is hard to do.

To make Principle #2 a real energy booster for your business, you also have to look beyond the top 5 people. If you take principle # 1 of serving and apply that serving mindset to everybody you encounter, your network will explode exponentially – provided you combine it with

**Principle #3: Give without Expectation of Return**

To attract relationships you need to be the one who is offering valuable gifts and services. Sometimes it is advice for a problem a new contact is describing to you. Sometimes it is a tool or resources you have and can share to help overcome an obstacle. Sometimes it is connecting one contact you have with another one that just joined your network. Sometimes it is giving something away without being paid because you know it helps even though the other person is currently not in a position to pay you.

It's strange how the universe works. When I changed my mindset, got back to giving and serving before receiving, and focused on the top 5 people as well as all the other relationships in my contact list and rolodex, requests started to come into my inbox and voicemail, almost daily.

Admittedly I needed to reactivate a lot of contacts that had sat dormant because I thought they would get to me if they needed me. When I began engaging, suddenly my relationships and my business success increased dramatically.

On this path it is important to remain aware of

**Principle #4: Honor Trust by Knowing what you Know**

This might sound a little cryptic. It goes back to what it means to be an expert. Fundamentally we have a tendency to put experts on a pedestal, initially for what we know they are an expert for, and then more and more for all issues that we believe the expert could know something about. A lot of people don't believe that they are an expert even if their friends, family and colleagues tell them all the time that they are. I am an expert in skill development for people who want to become better managers, leaders, communicators, and business owners. During the last 15 years I read hundreds of books about the topics that relate to these communities. I have received a lot of tools and techniques from these books and from companies that developed programs to help these groups.

Ultimately I began developing a number of my own tools. Here are just a few examples:

**PANDA** – a delegation technique
**MEDU** – a style and communication assessment that tells you what style you apply and how aligned it is with the way you communicate
**The Outcome Cycle** of Communication: a tool that allows you to conduct tricky and uncomfortable conversations i.e. for performance reviews or when a team member screwed up – and have a good outcome.
**Innovation Mapping** – an experiential approach to organization wide

issues and how to come up with new path forward that really get implemented

When you begin the transition from Beggar to having the Choice to select the projects, contracts, and people you want to work with, you will encounter opportunities where the reward is very tempting but you know in your heart that you are not an expert or, sometimes, know nothing about what is really needed to be successful.

In these situations it is important to realize that a contract you sign or an opportunity you choose is directly connected with the Trust that those who face the problem, issue or request your help, put into you. The best way you can honor that Trust is by accepting projects, opportunities and providing help from the deep knowing that you can actually help – that you know a path into the future that has a high probability of success. If you can't honestly say that to yourself know how to proceed, don't choose the project or opportunity.

I know it can be hard, especially when the reward, financially or otherwise, is very tempting. What has helped me to overcome the initial disappointment of rejecting an offer is the old statement from Peter Drucker, the business guru, who said: (paraphrased): "It can easily take you years to develop a trusting relationship and reputation – and sometimes seconds to ruin it"! When I look at that risk, it is easier to reject a choice and know that the relationship and the trust in you is intact. With that in mind, we get to

**Principle #5: Under-Promise and Over-Deliver**

When you have decided to accept an offer or choice, it is very important to identify what the expectations are. What does the customer really look for? What would be a great result? I suggest developing a set of questions that I call "The Fairy Dust Experiment". You are asking your interested client to describe what the outcome at the end of your involvement, initiative or project would be, assuming that all the things that could be in the way (like money, tools, time, etc.) could be instantly blown away by fairy dust.

Now that you have that description in mind, you want to find ways to get to this described  outcome and a little more – sometimes even a lot more. Besides applying the Fairy Dust Experiment to get an idea about the desired outcome, you serve your effort and your client very well by also identifying milestones and sub-goals. This allows you to over-deliver on your path to the end-result. You will see that your clients love to be pleasantly surprised about what you provide. That deepens their trust in you, develops your reputation as a person or company, showing that every penny of investment is really worth it and one more thing:

Your clients love to tell people in their network about their success stories. When that starts happening, you get choices, projects, opportunities offered that you never anticipated.

I have been asked to change learning programs in a customized way resulting in the new program being contracted more often and for more money than the original course. I have been asked to coach people individually based on a leadership group retreat where the income from coaching was more than that of the retreat, and more importantly, these initial coaches still send me new people years after the original event.

You might be reading about this principle and ask yourself:

**"Well, that's great but what if the choices I am offered are all not really fitting into my wheelhouse or core competencies?"**

I suggest to "build bridges to your success" by applying

### Principle # 6: Collaboration beats Competition

With the advent of social media and the internet, we are all much more connected than we used to be. I could not do as much as I do all the time without help. Some of it is here in the United States, but I also have my 'right-hand-angle' in Pune, India. She is not just available for simple administrative tasks but has grown into a true associate whose ideas, input, and suggestions I value and who I trust to do a lot of the work I used to do myself. In many cases she does things better than I would – because we can both focus on applying principle #4 – she knows what she is good at and I know the same about myself - and together we are building a good team on specific projects for certain clients.

As mentioned earlier this principle can also serve as a bridge-builder when the offers you receive don't really fit your skillset – yet.

When you work actively on building relationships you can't avoid learning what people do, like, what they are good at, and what they love to do more of. As you build your network of experts, initially in your local area, then country wide, and potentially even beyond that, you learn more and more about your networks expertise. In my case we have experts in

Europe, South America, Middle-America, Australia, and the Middle East. – don't ask me why Asia has escaped us so far …!?!

These experts totally know that marketing themselves to gain business is a substantial effort and cost. If you have developed a relationship and offer an expert to share any of the offers and choices you have been presented with, they typically don't mind giving you some of the revenue that is generated. I don't call it a principle but an approach that has served me well in this collaborative process: "80% (sometimes 90%) of something is better than 100% of nothing – meaning giving a choice/opportunity that was presented to you – and you share it for a 20% (or 10%) referral fee, is definitely worth it.

Through this sharing activity I recently was able to accept a strategy project for a large French cosmetics company in New York. A friend of mine did the work in her neighborhood when it would have been thousands of miles of travel for me - and she did a better job than I could have ever done because it was right smack in the middle of her core competency. Besides the revenue for her and the referral fee for me, our relationship is much deeper now and, going forward, we will look for more projects like this.

In addition it has taught me a lot about strategy development and I would feel more comfortable to take on such a project would one come my way in my geographic area – it literally build a bridge to a new expertise I did not have before.

I could now honor the trust a company would put in me for such a project, and if needed, could always bring my friend from the East Coast in to help.

Collaborating this way (and in many other ways you can imagine), leads to a flood of relationships, connections, and project/contract offers.

With all these principles in mind the last one points us towards the attitude required to be able to look at your own path with a smile that comes from success:

### Principle #7: The glass is half-full

This last principle is probably more personal to me than the others before. Having been raised in Germany I could not escape the cultural imprint. This imprint teaches a fundamentally skeptical view on life. If you present a problem of any kind to a German, naturally we are able to immediately and without hesitation, create a long list of all the things that stand in the path of success. Everything that could go wrong is listed. Any imaginable (and in some cases unimaginable) negative aspect that can be identified will be identified.

After a while of analyzing an idea, proposition, issue, challenge, or problem, the originally neutral starting point is completely covered with a mountain of negativity that makes it obvious that success is virtually impossible.

I had to learn that this approach makes live and business success much harder than it needs to be.

Experts call this behavior the "glass half empty"-attitude. Half of the glass if filled with problems that could be listed and the remaining space is probably there for more problems and issues that have not yet been identified. They work with the "Obstacle – Glass".

I believe to be successful you need to have a "glass half full" attitude. You need to work with the "Opportunity-Glass" In this case the glass is already filled with half of what you need to be successful. It is not filled with problems but with opportunities, tools, tips, tricks, techniques and things you can do.

Bottom line is this: If you have the "glass half-full" attitude, all you need to do is find a few more things to add to what's already in place to turn an opportunity into a success. You can say: "There is something in place I can build on!"

Stay away from people with the glass half empty view – all they are looking for are more problems they can find to fill the Obstacle-Glass. Then they have to develop solutions to get all the problems and obstacles out of the glass to make room for opportunity. In most cases they deem that to be too hard to do and they end up doing nothing or looking for others to take action first.

If the Opportunity-Glass is already half full and you can add something positive to it, something you know or have expertise in, go for it, and apply yourself.

For those cases where your contribution is only small, find others in your network you can share the opportunity with. That will breed success.

As you are supporting that Opportunity-Glass/project, others will appear where you can be the lead and your contacts help you.

Previous projects become bridges to new opportunities. As your network grows you will have to make choices about what you like to be involved in and what you share with others, and – sometimes, what you reject – which will be a strange feeling at first.

Just recognize those few cases as a sign of your success and a good reason to ask yourself: How did I get here? – it will encourage you to share your journey with others so they can learn from you.

If you like to learn more about my journey, feel free to contact me or take a look at: http://www.AxelMeierhoefer.com

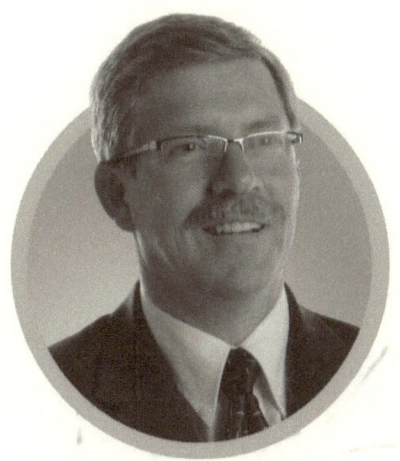

**Dr. Axel Meierhoefer**

Dr. Axel, has a PhD in Leadership and a Master's Degree in Organizational Management. He completed a 22 year career as an aviator in the Air Force, followed by executive experience in the IT industry and then founded his first company. By now he has evolved into a professional facilitator and lecturer.

Axel has been leading his main company AKC LLC for the last 10 years and founded 4 other companies that operate successfully. In an environment with increasing complexities Axel and his team focus on program management, skill development, and individual support through mentoring, coaching, and speaking. With increasing demands on teams, he is helping organizations, executives, leaders, and their team members through facilitation, sales training, talent & leadership development, communication improvement and conflict management. Clients span from small businesses and entrepreneurs to Fortune 100 clients like Boeing, Bayer, Cisco, Johnson & Johnson, GE, Verizon, and Merck.

# 9

## PIECE OF CAKE

### - BY FRANKIE MOONEY, MOTIVATIONAL SPEAKER AND AUTHOR OF 'TEENAGE ENTREPRENEUR: SECRET OF SUCCESS'.

Please be aware: The contents of this chapter have been written in such a way that may appear to be grammatically incorrect. This is by design and is written in such a way so as to accelerate the learning process. Written hypnotically to ensure key learning's are not filtered by the conscious mind. The conscious mind is the mind that is reading this right now where as your unconscious mind remains responsible for the 'background operations' like your breathing, blinking and understanding of core concepts at a deeper level. Relax comfortably and read this chapter with profound sense of curiosity as though the next word on the page you read may be the answer to a puzzle you have been eager to solve. Nonetheless reading the chapter in and of itself and in it's entirety will be enough to equip you with the insights and tools your unconscious mind will need to help you where you need it and when you need it most. This chapter has been engineered to directly program your unconscious through sophisticated use of various anecdotes, analogies and imagery presented in a specific format to allow the ideas to bypass critical thinking faculties. You will find your thinking and behavior will change in the direction you find most preferable in relation to what it is you want to do. If you do not notice changes know that this is ok and your unconscious will be making the appropriate changes it needs to allow your conscious mind to think and behave as it prefers.

The book Norwegian Wood by Haruki Murakami, first published in Japanese in 1987, and in English in 1989, has the following: "Just remember, life is like a box of chocolates." ... "You know, they've got these chocolate assortments, and you like some but you don't like others? And you eat all the ones you like, and the only ones left are the ones you don't like as much? I always think about that when something painful comes up. "Now I just have to polish these off, and everything'll be OK.' Life is a box of chocolates." It later appeared in the 1994 film Forrest Gump, when the lead character Forrest Gump (played by Tom Hanks) says "Mama always said life was like a box of chocolates. You never know what you're gonna get."

Etymology of a great quote and magnificent film aside, I would say life is a lot like cake. That goes for life, success, your destiny or anything else you might be in pursuit of attaining or mastering in one's time – it's a lot like a cake. Because you know with a cake a lot of people might look at it and they might adore it, crave it, lust after it even and when they finally take a bite they love it, you know? That big round brown sponge base with yellow cream topping and white icing sprinkled with all those little pink marshmallow pieces or they might hate it. For those who love it, whose noses open wider and lungs breathe in deeper to catch the full smell of the strawberry or chocolate when they see it again they know what to expect. It will never deviate. It is what it is and that individual knows what it is. For those who hate it, they never taste it again, give it another look or let the idea of eating it cross their mind again. The experience of that cake will never deviate.

Only when you understand what goes into how that cake is made can you change the cake. Know the ingredient and you can change the size, shape, color, even the taste. The person who knows how the cake is made can change the outcome of the cake for themselves and for others.

Now, I'm not a proponent of get rich quick schemes. If you're looking to make a serious amount of money fast but not interested in doing any work or putting in any effort for your information I won't be providing any formula's to break Wall Street or systems to clean out casinos. If that's what you're looking for from this chapter I won't disappoint you, you can contact me at my private email because I've got some really great magic beans that will work for you, and they're only $10. Who says money doesn't grow on trees, right?

However, for those of you, like me, who prefer a more holistic approach to life, business, success, prosperity, relationships, consciousness expansion and heart centered living then this chapter is designed for you.

For those of you familiar with the term NLP, just so you know so am I. I first got heed of this notion when I read an article about how world President's like Barack Obama and other leading politicians had been trained in Neuro Linguistic Programming to better communicate effectively. Those big brands like McDonalds had utilized the technology of NLP's subliminal communication models to enhance their advertising and better target consumers. Some noted it was 'mind control'. Whooa! "Mind Control" buzzy uh? Well I worked day and night to save enough money to go to London to meet the creator of this Mind-boggling technology and learn NLP. I had the options available to learn nlp from the person who learned nlp from the person who knew the guy who created it but being reminiscent of playing 'whisper down the lane' (Broken Telephone in the US) where the original intended message differs the further away from the source it gets whether due to erroneous corrections, anxiousness, impatience or people who just want to deliberately alter the intended information to guarantee a changed message by the end, lead me quite quickly to decide to train with the original creator and I'm glad I did as over the years I've met hundreds of people who seem to have digested the big book of nlp techniques but have no deep understanding of what it means for us as human beings living on this planet.

At age 18, I was the youngest licensed NLP master practitioner and when I returned from London, people asked me what I could tell them about it and I summed it up like this; If you don't take control of your mind, someone else will. NLP was an education. I was lucky to have learned it the way it was intended, at such a young age. Not only did it help me understand how our brains work & how our sense of sight, smell, touch and what we hear help create our experience of life but also opened the flood gates on my understanding of the structure of reality.

The mind is certainly one thing I took a great interest in understanding. If there is going to be anything in life I'm going to be spending a lot of time with, it's my mind, so I thought it best that I get to know it!

Many who know me will know I am an enthusiast of the martial arts. I enjoy learning about and studying all types of styles and different arts. It is equally important to develop and nurture the mind as it is to take care of the physical body. It's great to expand consciousness, connect with your greater mind and get high on life but remember when you fall back to earth your physical body needs to be well enough to handle impact. I have trained in ninjitsu for as long as I can remember. Let it be known that the days of old where ninja would creep the night aloof and unknowing, prone and ready to eliminate their target are gone and has since been swapped with the concrete jungles of today with its skyscrapers, cut-throat business practices and myriad guises of social-chameleonism.

In the book Essence of Ninjutsu by Masaaki Hatsumi, published in 2000 there is a beautiful quote that I have included here "I believe that Ninpo, the highest order of Ninjutsu, should be offered to the world as a guiding influence for all martial artist. The physical and spiritual survival methods eventually immortalized by Japan's ninja were in fact one of the sources of Japanese martial arts. Without complete and total training in all aspects of the combative arts, today's martial artist cannot hope to progress any further than mere proficiency in the limited set of muscular skills that make up his or her training system. Personal enlightenment can only come about through total immersion in the martial tradition as a way of living. By experiencing the confrontation of danger, the transcendence of fear of injury or death, and a working knowledge of individual personal powers and limitations, the practitioner of Ninjutsu can gain the strength and invincibility that permit enjoyment of the flowers moving in the wind, appreciation of the love of others, and contentment with the presence of peace in society." So if you ever fancy a go at martial arts, search for your local Bujinkan organization, it'll only cost you $20 and you'll have a blast! The skills you can learn through the martial arts will incorporate into your life and benefit you in ways that you cannot imagine.

Everything is connected. From the first paragraph about NLP to the second paragraph about martial arts and going deeper now, the very reason you have acquired this book and reading this chapter and if and when you further your learning of the structure of reality and I strongly recommend you do, think like me, perhaps using The Holographic Universe as a starting point you will quickly come to this insightful understanding. Now, a lot of people when they come across sayings like "It's all an illusion", "everything is a hologram", "nothing exists" they feel a little helpless and some eventually worship volcanoes or worst, they lose the ability to make things fun. The deep learning outcome from the teachings of the structure of reality and what it has to tell you is that it offers you the opportunity to investigate and understand the relationship between you and reality. There is a fantastic film called What The Bleep Do We Know (the link I have included at the end of this chapter) that utilizes amazing visuals to illustrate the unseen forces at work in our reality. As always I only intend to point to various truths I have discovered that have given me insight and whether you decide to investigate those further and discover if those are truths for you also and should the ideas I raise resonate with you on any level, I suggest you do research those further, the choice is and always will be yours to make.

Any project I have ever undertaken has been because I thought I could do it better than what I had seen done previous. If I could innovate, re-invent, develop, enhance or in any shape or form make it better than what was available I would do it. That and the unyielding feeling of excitement for an idea is a proponent of getting things done. The excitement is one of the most important things that carries me through from initial planning and development to execution and completion.

I remember seeing something, whether it was in person, on the TV, in a magazine or somewhere else and thinking "I can do that". It was then followed up with "How can I do that?" and the journey into finding the ingredients of such an endeavor would begin. In my early teens I vividly remember aspiring to be the next Richard Branson, entrepreneur extraordinaire, the next Paul McKenna world renowned hypnotist and the next Tony Robbins world famous life coach and healer. Aspiring and modeling these people really did help me get to do things extraordinary but really appreciating and encouraging my self is what got me through the plateaus in life.

As a speaker in schools I would get asked lots of questions. Even today I still get asked a lot of questions and if I am to think about it and tell you what question I get asked the most it's "How do you do that?" which is quite fitting for this book, don't you think? I could go on and on giving you various anecdotes and that alone could fill an anthology in itself but you know, deeper still the real problem these people were and still do experience is that they were seeking the permission. They were looking for the permission to go live the life of their dreams, the permission to do the thing they really wanted to do. Are you seeking the elusive permission slip? In their heads they have so many reasons why NOT to go ahead and try something (one of the main things I always do is focus on the one reason why I should do something and none of the billions of other reasons why not to), usually due to hearing negative things for too long and having learned lots of bad habitual thinking habits ("Faulty Programming") "What will it say about me?" and other negatively reinforced thoughts that are taught subliminally to the unconscious (and sometimes conscious!) by friends, family and society regardless of their good intentions. There is a particularly funny scene In The Simpsons episode "The Day The Violence Died" (Season 7), where the creation of Itchy & Scratchy cartoons is disputed and the joke I like is included here for you; "But so what? Animation is built on plagiarism. If it weren't for someone plagiarizing The Honeymooners we wouldn't have The Flintstones. If someone hadn't ripped off Sergeant Bilko, there'd be no Top Cat. Huckleberry Hound? Chief Wiggum? Yogi Bear? Ha! Andy Griffith. Edward G. Robinson. Art Carney. Your Honor, you take away our right to steal ideas where are they gonna come from- her?" Marge responds, "Uh- hmm- How 'bout Ghost Mutt?" Now I am not saying go out and copy someone else's work, not at all. Not unless you enjoy lawsuits and missing out on the satisfaction of deriving your own work, but because someone else has done something (whether that be a great scientist, thinker, entrepreneur, leader, etc.) doesn't mean you cannot be too or get involved in the same line of work as someone you admire or look up to out of fear that you might be considered "like them" or "copying them". In most cases these people are living examples that you too can live the life you want to. Understand that no-one is like you, you are the only one of you, unique with infinite potential to live the life of your dreams (whatever those may be). So if its permission to do something you need, let me give it to you. Its ok for you to live the life of your dreams. To plan, pursue and achieve any goal you should so desire, regardless of what anyone else (friends, parents, extended family, peers or others) may think. It is of no concern to you what they think. This is your life and you have my permission to live it fully, honestly and authentically. It's alright to be your unique self and express the multifaceted personality that you are. But use your common sense, I'm not saying go start operating in a medical centre as a surgeon without obtaining the relevant training and qualifications. As for Ghost Mutt? There is a thrilling rap-induced movie called Ghost Dog:Way of The Samurai (1999) starring Forest Whitaker in one of his best films as lead as 'Ghost Dog' who's psychological and spiritual state is worth checking out.

I want to connect with those of you who read and study about pursuing those ambitions, reaching those goals, 'getting success' and feel kind of cornered by the idea that never mind 'how did you do it' but 'how do you work out what you want to do?' and I want you to approach the investigation of how you work out what it is you want to do with this idea and the idea is that Life is a hallway and at the end is your destiny. Free Will is how you choose to travel through that hallway. You can walk, run, hop, skip, crawl, whatever you like, you have control and it's your choice. Undoubtedly, you will reach your destiny.

I navigate life's highs and lows as they come. I pursue projects and ideas that are full of inspiration and excitement as much as I can and that offer me an opportunity to continue the creative process of the universe, something the universe has done before me and will continue to do so long after I'm gone. Following my passions and being in 'the flow', appears to lead me to meetings, chance encounters and synchronicities that relate and further develop & enhance my life. I take solace in the idea that I often experience my thoughts and not my circumstances and, understanding that what I feel may not be rooted in actual reality, I feel my feelings nonetheless as part of my experience as I know, soon like a dark cloud on a summers day it will pass and the sun will shine again and ultimately know the ultimate truth that regardless of what clouds may come, just above them is a sky that is free from storms and this thought should remind you that peace is ever prevalent and only ever a thought away.

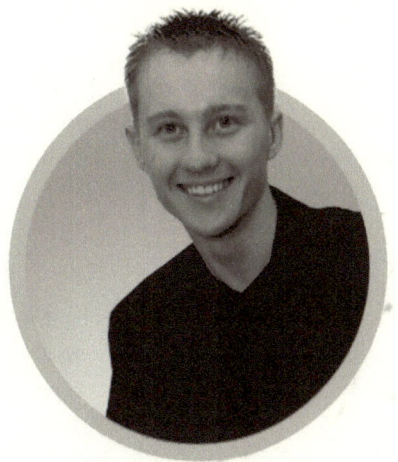

**Frankie Mooney**

Frankie Mooney is Founder and CEO of 5051 Worldwide, a multinational company specializing in various industries. Founded in 1997 as an integrated e-commerce, music and sports entertainment company, 5051 has been researching and developing it's various businesses for over a decade and now boasts an impressive portfolio of companies including a multi-award winning digital, technical and creative agency, record label, publishing house, digital new media group, professional wrestling federation and a complete in-house development and training suite.

Frankie Mooney is an entrepreneur, web developer, motivational speaker and author of 'Teenage Entrepreneur: Secret of Success'. He has kickstarted and grown multiple online ventures, promotes live events and hosts seminars and workshops.

With over 15 years experience as an internet entrepreneur, Frankie provides individuals and businesses with expert advice in website design, search engine optimization, ecommerce and internet marketing and provides professional hosting, email and technical support solutions.

Frankie is a licensed master practitioner of Hypnosis & NLP through the Society of NLP and was trained by the creator of Neuro Linguistic Programming, Dr Richard Bandler. He was also trained by Paul McKenna, John La Valle & Kathleen La Valle and continues to learn from teachers and mentors including Hollywood Supercoach Michael Neill.From his Glasgow clinic, Frankie provides personal coaching and can help you if you want to quit smoking, lose weight, rid yourself of any fears or phobias, reduce your stress or increase your confidence.

Frankie is an enthusiastic martial artist & professional wrestler and has trained in many disciplines. He currently provides authentic martial art training, fitness and combat conditioning through his exclusive Warrior Spirit programs. He is Director of professional wrestling federation UPW Live (www.upwlive.com) and professional wrestling training institute, Slam School (http://slamschool.co.uk).

Frankie has a strong philosophy of giving back to the community and in 2003 launched the Scottish Executive's enterprise in education initiative 'Determined To Succeed' with First Minister Jack McConnell as well as Make Your Mark and other young enterprise initiatives locally and internationally. 10 years on the Lifelong Learning Strategy continues to form part of education syllabus.

Links:

www.5051worldwide.com
www.frankiemooney.com
www.facebook.com/imfrankiemooney
www.twitter.com/frankie_mooney
www.uk.linkedin.com/in/frankiemooney

What The Bleep Do We Know
https://www.youtube.com/watch?v=ioONhpIJ-NY

# 10

## FINDING THAT ELUSIVE POT OF GOLD AT THE END OF THE RAINBOW OR DID YOU SAY YOU WANT SOME GOLD?

- BY DANIEL VAN NIEKERK, LICENSED FINANCIAL ADVISOR.

There are 3 kinds of people in life: Those who MAKE things happen, those who sit by WATCHING things happen, and those who wake up one day wondering ;"What the HECK happened??"

Times were tough in South Africa for us as a family in 2007.

I spent 15 years in our family musical instruments business MusicFest SA, and was looking for a change. Amongst other things, I am a bass player and musician and with old friend Michael Naranjo started a hard rock group called ONE DAY REMAINS.(ODR)

Things looked up for ODR, I managed to secure a record deal with a good South African record label David Gresham Records, and the Rock, touring and gigging life style kicked in full force – concerts, music videos, recording, TV slots…the whole 9 yards. Famous as last !

Those who are married will know that this rock & roll life style and marriages are not always the best of friends, and being a family guy I had to make the right decision – family over fame.

I left ODR, was out of the retail game after 15 years --- NOW what?

With affirmative action being the way it is in South Africa, a guy my age (39) and race was not really the flavour of the month and so work was really hard to find…I had to improvise.

Various work experiences that included luxury property sales, right down to driving a Taxi in St Francis Bay in the Eastern Cape lead me to respond to an advertisement to work in offshore financial services in Botswana.

After a successful interview with the proprietor in Sandton Johannesburg, a short induction phase and training followed in Gaborone Botswana, and a few weeks later I was on a plane to start my new career as a trainee offshore financial advisor --- Tanya and our two then-small boys Luc and Logan  was to stay in South Africa for the time being until I got settled.

I was always good in sales & client services, having been in retail for 15+ years…so this was something I could really sink my teeth into.

Little did I know that this course of action was to put my young family and I through the most challenging times of our lives !

Being thrown in the deep side of the pool, I was to see my first prospect 20mins after landing at Gaborone airport – wow. This is not always a bad thing, but as I developed, I realised that I do NOT want to be just some commission jocky or policy salesperson...I actually really care about people and what they really need.

I often objected to the archaic "old-school" style-, hard-closing sales techniques used in our industry, and as it so often happens with those of us who advocate positive change, it also made me unpopular with some people in the industry.

Let's be honest, some people just don't like the boat rocked --- enters 15 years seasoned consumer advocate Daniel van Niekerk, shaking the trees trying to see what falls out.

I was doing fairly good sales, I wrote the 1st piece of business amongst my intake as a rookie IFA, and with the encouragement of my manager managed to move Tanya & the kids over to Gaborone.

I was a social media and new media freak, and my "boss" just not see any value in pursuing a formidable online presence, advertising in local publications as this "did not fit the image of the company" he would reiterate.

I've done this kind of online marketing successfully throughout my decade or so tenure at Musicfest SA in South Africa and got my band a major record deal using this very skillset --- what do you MEAN it doesn't work? I was a SEO champ, qualified web developer...graphic designer, I could DO stuff.

Well, social media was blocked at the office and although I could've circumvented all of these measures if I really wanted to, I just felt like I was in ship going nowhere slowly – Look, I loved what I did (and still do to this day) , it was never a job to me, but I wanted MORE out of this career than just seemingly flogging savings policies.

I started looking around and eventually fixed my eye on South East Asia. I communicated with a few offshore IFA firms, and managed to impress enough to secure a few long distance phone interviews.

After one particularly good call with MD Mark Payne in Singapore, I was invited for a come-look-see-decide trip and the company offered to pay for my Hotel Stay in Singapore.

I jumped on a plane around October 2010 (over a long weekend) to go and meet Mark and his team. I had did some online psychometric tests, had to draw up a business plan and 2 days later I had an offer of employment from a prestigious IFA firm in hand --- AWESOME.

The company wanted me to start asap, ideally that November of 2010 already, but after crunching the numbers Tanya and I realised that I might be a bit too much too soon. Singapore as beautiful as it is, is NOT cheap and another major family move so relatively soon after just settling them in Botswana was just too expensive in the end.

I was not going to leave them again for 6 months like I had to before, so it's either all of us or no-go.

Little did I realise that a certain individual was opening my mobile phone bill (which came to the Botswana office), and probably checked through my emails as well, although I can't prove this.

So as to not rip open old wounds, suffice to say that this individual turned Spies R Us / Commando on me and before long I was called into the usual  monthly review meeting , which ended up being a "Kangaroo Court" session interrogating me about looking around at other firms. I was "caught out" – HA !

Apparently it's a crime to look for better opportunities elsewhere and leave that company --- Sound familiar to some out there?

I was summarily dismissed (illegal by the way), my phone sim card taken from me (also illegal), the old 2nd hand company laptop I used was removed from my office WHILE I was in the "review meeting", the car pool keys repossessed and  my office raided FBI style, just like in the movies !

My "crime?" Looking for a better opportunity where I could apply myself more.

The actual ensuing story is quite long and detailed, I don't have the space to go into the particulars here, but I was given the value of $20 in Botswana currency, and told something that uses that letter that comes after "E" in the alphabet.

So:  No money = no rent & no school fees, no transport, limited money for food whilst we had a rented  house full of furniture bought 2 months before…JEEPERS !

Oh yes…and to add insult to injury…just to make things a liiiiiiiiltle more interesting, I got pick pocked the same day – SO no wallet either.

We were literally stranded in a foreign country, my still-pending work permit due from the office of the President (any day now- at that time) cancelled immediately out of pure spite. The official reason given to the labour department for the permit cancellation? :- I couldn't do the job !? --- We were now officially on overstay because the staff were told not to renew our last work waivers since our work permits were due to come out soon and would override the expired temporary work permits.

We had to pay a fine for "overstay", which was exactly what said person wanted to achieve. He actually said to me that he would like to have me deported ! What a sad, twisted individual.

While this maddening persecution and chaos ensued, I somehow managed to connect with another IFA company in Bangkok and secured an offer of employment based on the Singapore offer. The cost of living in Thailand was considerably less than Singapore so it was DO or DIE. Returning to South Africa was just not an option.

To make a long story a bit shorter (nothing short of movie script stuff, no less) we exited or "escaped" Botswana literally with the clothes on our backs after a mediocre short notice garage sale. We sold most of our household items bought only two months before at a 1/3 of the price or less in order to buy plane tickets out of there.

Some personal items we had to leave in storage…which ended up being a 3-year storage excrcise costing 50 times the actual value of the personal items like photo albums, family videos, keep sakes and other irreplaceable items…but that is a story for another time. We all slept on the floor the last 2 days in Botswana.

We felt like criminals…having to" escape" Botswana --- you know like in the movies when you approach the customs / emigration officials and they take that extra long time to go through your passport, frowning…squinting their eyes, holding it up to compare the photo likeness (I probably looked like an emotional wreck !), then scanning the document, looking at me…as if you're a wanted felon trying to escape justice and something does not quite add up. I'm telling you…it was just like that.

Taking off the runway was a HUGE relief….we MADE it…feeling like bank robbers sighing a sigh of relief as they depart for Rio de Janeiro --- only thing is, we never did anything wrong.

We really loved living in Bangkok, but again had to move down South to Huahin (Prachuap Khirikhan) after the 2011 floods, a news story covered world-wide at the time over a few weeks – Phew, moving and moving…AGAIN.

After a further year of some normalcy, now living in paradise,1km from a secluded beach (Hat Sai Noi) in Kao Thao just outside HuaHin, Africa beckoned…this time Uganda. I was headhunted by IFA Match to join a major IFA firm out in rural Africa.

Why leave paradise? Well, I guess after 3 years of home schooling, - running around in nothing more than their underwear most of the time, the kids felt a bit lonely as our immediate area did not have a lot of "farang" (foreigner) kids, and they needed friends.

I thought it best to have the family stay where they are for a while (there are worst places to be left alone for a while I guess !), so I can go do my thing.

Well, well, well…I am FROM Africa, but rural Africa is another story. Sure, I was a military guy, I went to the Navy…I can easily rough it for a while..which I did amongst other things…which is ALSO a story for another time.

Well, its the end of 2013, its almost a YEAR since left Thailand.

My advanced social media and networking skills secured me two national TV appearances talking on NTV Uganda about savings and investments – FREE advertising for me, the Uganda CEO Magazine, the RedPepper, NewVsion all queuing to print some of my financial banter & educational material I send out to my 8000+ local audience and my 17 000+ International network.

Awesome, the "Muzungu" (white man / wonderer I am known as by many here) is becoming somewhat of a local celebrity in Uganda…famous, AGAIN ! haha

Well, Tanya and the kids understandably still felt isolated in Thailand, with dad gone again to find something that will work for the family in the long term.

I still had to become properly "legal" in Uganda, being a long term repeat visitor for all practical purposes at that time. I just could not settle them in Uganda under such insecure circumstances. Perhaps if it was our first move, you know…a bit of an adventure, but after the Botswana saga there was no way I'd allow the slightest possibility of anything like that to

EVER happen to them again.

I didn't want to just trip in and out all the time, as many IFA's do, I wanted to plug in and I really fell in love with the place...GREAT weather all year round, an endless summer, but very alone without my family. I was a very involved father since birth, so there are days I just cried for them, missing them so much. A year is a long, long time...and money was in short supply despite my media presence etc. and I was essentially self-employed ploughing away in a nation with no savings culture, and where $300 was the average salary.

WHY on earth do that and not go to Middle East, or China like the rest of the herd?

Well, I would hope by now you'd appreciate that I like doing things differently...I saw massive, massive potential.

I had a tough time convincing the foreign IFA firm to put down roots in Uganda...to incorporate, so I can apply for a proper work & residence permit....so this kept me away from my not-so-little-anymore ones and Tanya even longer. Delays upon delays and eventually the IFA company decided to re-focus their apatite in a more reliable jurisdiction. We parted on very good terms and Africa was just not really what they were after.

It was decided to move Tanya and the kids back to South Africa, primarily for schooling reasons, while I try and sort out what must have seemed like quite a mess...seemingly no direction, not able to get settled.

Back to offshore recruiter IFA Match and BD Wealth Management expressed interest in my activities in Uganda.

BD Wealth Co-owner Alan Dempster, Zimbabwean born, had a very successful financial services career for many years in South Africa after fleeing the Mugabe regime in Zimbabwe and later settled in Kuwait with his wife who is a British national.

Alan and business partner Olly runs what is known as probably the most successful expat IFA company in Kuwait.

It was time to incorporate in Uganda...FINALLY -- after a year living in exile, so to speak, with my own country having nothing to offer me, and I mean NOTHING.

Could 2015 be the year I can re-unite our family, the family I never thought I'd ever have to seemingly abandon ?

Then something happened that changed our lives forever…something that put a BIG YES answer to the question before this sentence.

A Ugandan friend of mine introduced me to KaratBars International.

Karatbars is an E-commerce business in 123 countries and helps people all over the world save physical GOLD (Karatbar gold Cards – the new "Global Money") in small increments.

This is gold  for the masses, the best gold  at the best price. There is also an opportunity to generate a substantial, passive, residual income by referring others to the program.

The best thing is that you can register a FREE, worldwide, online, -gold account with no cost to join and no set-up or registration fees. There are no monthly quotas or requirements or "autoship's" etc.

Well, I was NOT looking to get involved in some MLM scheme selling pills & powders, toothpaste, lotions and stuff.  Tanya and myself dabbled in MLM's 10years ago back in South Africa, so I had my fill of hype…the garage full of expiring consumable diet shakes and supplements we almost eventually had to give away.

But GOLD?….this was really something unique and interesting ! Who hates gold…right? Everybody wants it, but very few people can afford bricks of the shiny stuff…including me.

As a financial advisor, the whole concept  just made absolute sense ! Buy small increments of a 5000+ year old commodity that always appreciates: Change paper currency for REAL money and thereby protect your wealth and financial future ! A fantastic affordable hedging strategy—WOW !

With gold up almost 4000% since 1971 (at time of this publication), I felt that this is something I could actually sink my teeth into.

The business side of it is totally optional and is for  those who want to work the network marketing side of it. Some people just want to buy gold outright, so that's great. The business side is a system of getting paid for introducing others to the program…no rocket science here, we introduction commission in the offshore IFA industry as well.

Karatbar gold is 999.9 pure 24K LBMA certified, London good delivery currency grade...you know, the GOOD stuff -- not the cheap jewellery, gold coins stuff you can buy down the road. This is the gold grade you find stored in places like Fort Knox.

With less than 1% of the world population owning gold, the market potential is HUGE !

This will be the largest market transfer in world history.

Over 1.4 QUADRILLION DOLLARS Fiat Paper Money Market transferring to Gold, Silver and Oil Backed Money... GLOBALLY

When Karatbars expands to 1/3 of just 1% of that Market Transfer...it will BE BIGGER THAN ALL MARKETS of  Health, Wellness, Weight Loss, Nutrition, Water, Food, Juice, Coffee, Energy Drinks, Beauty, Jewelry, Gifting, Shopping Portals, Services, Penny Auctions, Advertising, Cars, Shoes, Travel And Clothes...

COMBINED !

Now tell me that isn't awesome !

Karatbar rules prohibit me from quoting the 6-7 figure incomes we earn, but if you want to know more about an opportunity that has changed lives GLOBALLY...something that is not just some fad, or passing fashion...then   you   need   to   visit   my   website   at http://www.financialadvisoruganda.com for more info.

So, from having to LEAVE our home country due to affirmative action, to moving to Africa being persecuted by a real twisted ex-boss who was hell-bent on ruining my career and good standing (just because he thought he could !) just for leaving his company...narrowly escaping the continent to start over in SE Asia with the clothes on our backs...and BACK to rural East Africa dodging Ebola, Malaria, Yellow Fever, fighting off bedbug infestations, even terrorists at some point !! What a roller coaster ride and how to tables have turned....and Uganda is fantastic, I wouldn't go back to South Africa permanently ever.

And THAT ladies and gentleman is HOW I DID IT !

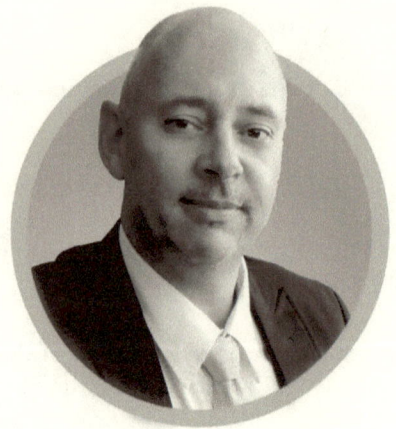

**Daniel Van Niekerk**

Licenced Financial Advisor representing BD Wealth Management in Uganda, specialising in offshore financial planning for expats and Africans across Africa.

**Company Website:** www.bd-wm.com
**Personal Business –** KaratBars International Affiliate
**Affiliate ID:** https://www.karatbars.com/landing/?s=princedaniel
**Website:** http://www.financialadvisoruganda.com
**LinkedIn:** http://ug.linkedin.com/in/financialadvisorafrica
**Twitter:** https://www.twitter.com/ugandaadvisor
**Facebook :** https://www.facebook.com/totheairport

**Google+**
https://plus.google.com/u/0/+DanielDctorQROPSvanNiekerk/posts

**Daniel on Uganda NTV:**

· https://www.youtube.com/watch?v=qTQ5UO7lMTw
· https://www.youtube.com/watch?v=_ok3M7OLhIs

**Why now is a GREAT time to get into Gold:**

· https://www.youtube.com/watch?v=ut93jA-49xU

# HERE'S HOW I DID IT!

· https://www.youtube.com/watch?v=Upbrhw-Q9DI
· https://www.youtube.com/watch?v=HnDL6OBfAlQ

# 11

## MY JOURNEY TO WHOLENESS - I HAVE A NEED TO SOAR TO FEEL FULL IN MY CORE

- BY ELLIE BORDEN, A NATURAL LEADER, ENTREPRENEUR, LIFE AND BUSINESS COACH.

Have you discovered what fuels your decisions? Do you agree that emotions and desires guide our life's path? Do you envision your passion and life's dreams in vivid color and depth — vibrant and massively sized like you're seeing them on an IMAX screen? Do the sounds make you elated; give you butterflies; make you want to happy-cry? Do you truly believe that having a deeply rooted, emotionally-charged, dream is as important as executing the steps needed to achieve goals that are in line with that dream? I say, ABSOLUTELY. Emotionally driven goals are effortless motivators.

My dreams are never-ending and ever changing, and that is what has kept my spirit trekking through the hardest times. I find fulfillment in the journey itself. Adventure is something I value, and life gives me exactly that in response to my thirst for exploration. I stretch beyond my comfort zone and I am open to learning from human interaction and failed attempts. I want to give 1000% into everything I do, and I am a strong believer that everything in our universe is energy. Otherwise, it's business as usual. But, I think normal is boring, and so I chose to live in an extraordinary way instead. Here's how I did it.

I'm a Serial Entrepreneur, Business and Personal Development expert, and Keynote Speaker. I've been an Entrepreneur since my McGill University graduating year in 1999, when my husband and I opened a record shop at the young age of twenty one. About eighteen months later, while running our second company, a Marketing and Promotion Firm, I decided to also pursue my long time passion for music. Long story short, we signed a label deal with Ryko/Warner Brothers in NYC and released my first album in 2003. I've had the privilege to work with very successful and powerful people in the industry. I'm grateful to have met incredibly influential business people, performers, artists, and actors. What I love most about what I do now, as an expert speaker, is witnessing the powerful personal growth and empowerment of everyday people, and their experiences of everyday situations.

Looking back at the crucial moments that contributed to my success, what definitely stands out for me is purpose and passion. In 2005, I traded an action-packed NYC music career to start a family. We became pregnant the month after we left New York and I became one of the most meticulous, almost obsessed, conscientious "pregos" out there -- prenatal classes, 30+ books, herb lists to avoid, food lists, birth plans, and long lists of ingredients for my OBGYN to review. I became increasingly concerned when she hadn't heard of most of the ingredients in skin care products, hair products, general household products, and packaged foods that I was using and consuming. I have to admit that I grew increasingly frustrated and initially became very angry that there were so many hidden dangers in our everyday products—I felt like roaring from the rooftops like an enormous mama bear! Before this point, I thought that I was so "Eco-savvy," I had it all figured out. I recycled religiously, made healthy food choices, tried to always choose products that were eco-friendly and as natural as possible. What did I discover? I was in the "matrix" the whole time. Well, it was time to be unplugged, and I was ready to share knowledge that would let others decide for themselves: red pill or blue pill? I wanted freedom and clarity for my unborn baby. I needed to do everything in my power to carry a baby that was in as natural a state as possible—for a non-tampered chance at what was divinely designed for her.

I didn't know where I was going to start, or what my final vision really was. I just knew that I had to do something powerful! It didn't say much for my business plan at the time, because I never actually started out with one. I guess we could say that I followed a "snowball" business plan. It started small and became a giant boulder that sometimes felt like an avalanche — not something that I would recommend! Most of the time, I couldn't keep up with my own ideas and workload, so the snowball slowly grew into a firestorm of inspiration and hard work. It felt like a blend of "Mama Bear Syndrome" with a full cup of the "New York State of Mind." What I learned when I moved to Brooklyn for my music career, was that if you let a wasted minute go by in New York City you were already ten steps behind the eight ball. I loved the fast-paced hustle and bustle, and the creativity that poured out of me in those few years as a New Yorker. I am so thankful for my experience in the music industry—what a powerful one it was! It fit so well with my work ethic, and it allowed me to explore my boundaries and experiment how far I could push myself to excel. Everything I have created professionally and personally could not have been possible if that part of my life didn't exist. What an experience!

Putting the music industry behind me and while still focusing on my growing family, I dove into my new passion of contributing positively to a toxic-free world that regarded the value of women and children, and was against animal cruelty. It was so meaningful to me to be working on a brand that could educate and inspire other moms, and make it possible for their babies to also be healthier and learn about protecting our planet. I would work on my RawGoodies® brand for a few hours during the day, and once the kids were in bed, I would work some more while studying for my second passion at the time — towards a Coaching career. Once I had my second little girl, I had to face the fact that I wouldn't realistically be able to do everything "by the book," as I had my eldest about to start half-day preschool and a very busy husband away on business for long periods of time. BUT, then something happened that refuelled me during a horrible burnout. My eldest said "mommy I understand when you're busy because you're a superhero that helps and protects people..." Seriously??? I couldn't believe that she was perceiving my passions in that light. I was making a difference in her life that would stick with her forever! I couldn't give up, or roll over and be defeated by some hormones and exhaustion! My girls had the opportunity to witness something inspiring, and to learn that as long as they remain genuinely dedicated to the motivating factors that brought forth their dreams and aspirations, then they will naturally inspire more greatness in themselves and others.

It was a long four years of research and development. And then, RawGoodies® was a trademarked brand of eight collections with about three hundred products. The details of the actual process could easily fill an encyclopedia, with almost every tiny step having it's own share of drama and snags attached to it. However, each one of those steps lead to a celebration as well. What a moment it was when I officially launched with a "home party" weekend! Although I felt embarrassed that our website wasn't ready yet, my mom reminded me of all I had accomplished up to that point, and instructed me to look around the room—a complete boutique of hundreds of products sitting on display in my dining room! My mom would have to constantly remind me of my accomplishments along the way, as she's done all my life. We celebrated when I was ready to take my research to another level to the final creation, a tangible brand that would hopefully change lives and inspire change; we celebrated the creation of the names for every product; label designs; creation of each collection; getting the vanity number that we wanted "ECO-LOVE." There have been so many baby steps that gave way for many more baby steps. Every piece of the puzzle seemed to slowly fall into place.

Among all the sleepless nights, juggling career and family, and trying to have phone meetings while the two cubs were running around, as if it was Mardi Gras in our living room, I am very proud of where I am today. Today I see myself as a full woman with a fiery power-center that ignites critical thinking, passion, and empowerment. It has been a freakishly beautiful process of slow and steady growth that has been fuelled by the need to align my life's path with my values—uniqueness, creativity, adventure, leadership, equality, and justice. I continually strive for enlightenment and search for growth in wisdom-quests and self-reflection. Now excitedly enjoying a career as a Keynote Speaker, Business and Personal Development Expert, and having founded four very purposeful and fulfilling brands, I would encourage you to also find your deepest motivators and "always be dreaming." Our dreams give us purpose, help us grow, let us feel and share passion, drive us to inspire others to dream, and hopefully teach us that the lessons are in the details, and the true satisfaction of working to achieve our dreams is in the journey itself.

*Though the road's been rocky it sure feels good to me. -- Bob Marley*

## How do you envision *your* journey?

Would you say that you are a big dreamer when thinking about your future, your passions, and your visions of success? How about for your career, your dedication to the greater good, climbing the highest mountain, anything your heart desires? If you would say that you "dream big," do you see that dream in color when you envision it? Is it hazy, in neutral color patterns, or is it in vivid bright colors? Can you hear the sounds in this scene? Let's say you envision yourself leading a conference of scientist for a new cure. Can you hear the crowd of people clapping and do you feel warmth in your heart for your accomplishments and contributions? What really sets us apart when pursuing and reaching beyond our arm's length for our dreams? The more involved we make all of our senses, in the participation of the vision of our passions, the easier it is to stay motivated in the pursuit of these dreams.

Three things to ask yourself: How does what you're doing make you feel? Does it have a positive impact on others? Does it turn up the volume and increase the vibration of your life?

Are you having problems figuring out what your true passion is? 1. Ask yourself what makes your heart sing with excitement (music, community, animals, adventure)? 2. Identify your strengths and talents (have you gotten compliments on your patience, creativity, compassion)? 3. What are you passionate enough about that causes you effortless motivation? 4. Become proactive in your own life! Getting rid of victim mentality makes you feel in control, confident, and empowered. Those feelings open up possibilities and thus new passions.

What I encourage you to embrace is an awareness to the colors of your life's path. Learn your ABC's! Learn to *Adapt*, nurture *Balance*, and proceed with *Confidence*. Life is passionate for change and for a continuum of transformation — so in order to become fluid with the process you need to become passionate for what you will learn in every step of that change. Furthermore, embrace adversity, look adversity in the face and give it a GIANT smooch on the lips! You know what you say to tough times? You say "BRING IT ON -- BRING ON THE GROWTH, STRENGTH, EXPERIENCE, AND POWER." If you are prepared for curve balls, you'll bat them right out of the park every time. So, the advice I can give is that the best way to ride the wave is to be as fluid and formless as the water, no matter what your career path, passion, or dream may be. Gain as much practical knowledge and know-how, and also open your mind to what you can learn about yourself in the process. How can you be better today? Anything you don't get right today will be feedback for getting it right tomorrow.

One of the most important lessons that I've learned in my journey thus far is that you need the following equation for success in life, career, and business. Truth + Owning Truth = Actualizing Potential. Striving for a seamless partnership between finding your truth, as well as, owning that truth, enables you to approach decision making in a manner that is not distorted by limiting beliefs of self, fear of failure, or lack of passion. You must self-reflect and take accountability in order to be true to your emotional needs, shortfalls, passions, values, potential, and strengths. And, you must be proactive in standing tall in your truth—believing, tracing the lines of your imprint, leading, inspiring, sharing, living with transparent integrity, embracing self-love and respect.

**My secret — I consistently strive for a higher level of *emotional intelligence***

*Two Main Benefits of Higher Emotional Intelligence:*
People with higher emotional intelligence find it easier to form and maintain interpersonal relationships and to 'fit in' People with higher EIs are also better at understanding their own psychological state, this can include managing stress effectively and being less likely to suffer from depression and mood swings.

Studies have long shown that stress can have a lasting, negative impact on the brain. Exposure to even a few days of stress compromises the effectiveness of neurons in the hippocampus—an important brain area responsible for reasoning and memory. Weeks of stress cause reversible damage to neuronal dendrites (the small "arms" that brain cells use to communicate with each other), and months of stress can permanently destroy neurons. Stress is a formidable threat to your success—when stress gets out of control, your brain and your performance suffer.

*Three keys to developing a higher EI and healthier, more meaningful Relationships*

1. Inner Exploration: e.g. overcoming fears; eliminating blocks; stopping negative thinking and self-sabotage; identifying core values; cognitive distortions and limiting beliefs; overcoming victim mentality by building accountability and self-esteem; using "failure as an opportunity for growth.

2. Strategic planning and life-management: e.g. attaining laser focus; effortless motivation & drive; proper goal setting to match values; time-efficiency; plan business versus life.

3. Balance for happiness and inner peace: e.g. gaining control of your life; learn to let go; self-care; healthy lifestyle; stress management techniques; setting boundaries; mind and body connection work.

## Your Belief in *You*

You are in control of far more than you think. Your Belief in *You* is all you need to embark on any journey with your head held high. Confidence matters more than almost anything else in determining your success. And, mastering limitless confidence depends entirely on reprogramming your belief system. Therefore, zero in on a constructive thought process and belief system, embrace yourself as part of the universe and allow positive energy to flow through you, as well as, acknowledge that the process is the crucial factor to the end result. You can absolutely learn how to consciously create your reality. Our definition of reality is sometimes led by illusions, which leads to decision making that is motivated by a distorted perception, hence, self defeating thoughts and self-sabotage, and thus no growth. It helps me to envision the scene from the matrix here as well. Tapping into the vision of bending spoons with your mind, allowing energy to flow freely through all things. Once you make this second nature, you then have the power to mold and allow positive energy to flow through your entire being, and that of your environment, then there are no longer any blocks present. If our consciousness is powerful enough to collapse wave function in quantum physics experiments, and transform water crystals, then it is powerful enough to provide us with the ability to achieve what we truly desire.

### Final freeing thoughts

The most powerful thoughts for the pursuit of your potential:
-you have all of the skills and training necessary, or if you don't, you can acquire them.
-there is nothing holding you back from making different choices. Decision making can be empowering.
-you can let go of your doubt by eliminating your limiting beliefs and building your confidence.
-everything in your subconscious is composed of mental patterns and habits. Habits and mental patterns that block your growth can be replaced for ones that benefit it instead.

As you nurture your growth through inner exploration, strategies, and balance, you will naturally feel the alignment settling in "just right". That perfect feeling of calm, when even though the hardest times come along, your whole being automatically calculates the best suited lessons and the problem solving strategies to cope. You will no longer be reacting out of anger, frustration, sorrow, pain, excitement, boredom, happiness—that's what children do, as there emotional intelligence is underdeveloped. It is our absolute responsibility as adults to lead by example for our children, those close to us, and for the better good.

The most powerful internal force you possess is your own mind. Your reality is the subjective perception of your surroundings. Everyone perceives reality in his/her own way. What is experienced or observed is usually confined to the limits of beliefs of the observer. The most important thing is to be able to sacrifice what we are for what we could be. Make your journey about pushing the limits of your potential and get ready to Blaze Your Trail.

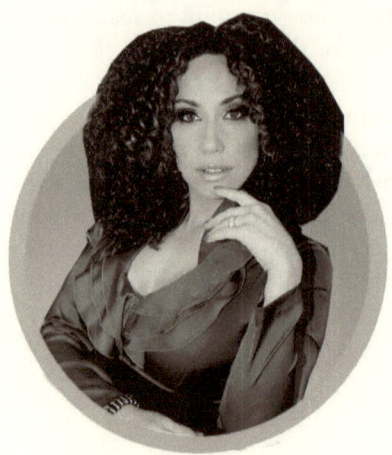

**Ellie Borden**

A natural leader, Entrepreneur, Life and Business Coach, and a sought after Keynote Speaker, Ellie's aim is to help people globally to become the leaders they are born to be. After graduating from McGill University, she operated a successful record shop.

Subsequently, her love of music led her to New York City, where she recorded music with world renowned artists like Swizz Beats, Just Blaze, Cool & Dre, Doug E. Fresh, Elephant Man, and more. After leaving the music industry to start a family, and inspired by motherhood, she hand-picked a research and development team to help her create the positive living brand, RawGoodies®. In 2009, perusing her passion to help others, she studied NLP and Feng Shui, and introduced the public to Blaze Your Trail — Life and Business Coaching.

Through her practice, Ellie encountered limitations in the confidence of many of her female clients; hence, Sexy Beast Lingerie was developed to push women's limits and enhance their sensuality. The Montreal Center for Anxiety and Depression recognized Ellie's stellar results in peak performance coaching, and she joined their "Dream Team," as their sole Life Coach/Personal Development Expert. A crucial element to Ellie's vision of the positive living experience, was to teach the winning combination of personal development and business training, thus the PowerCircle Women's Academy was established.

### Ellie Borden:

Main web: www.ellieborden.com
LinkedIn: https://www.linkedin.com/in/ellieborden
Main Email: ellieborden@icloud.com
Web: www.rawgoodies.com
FB:www.facebook.com/RawGoodies.Shop
Twitter: https://twitter.com/RawGoodies

### Blaze Your Trail Business & Life Coaching

Web: www.blazeyourtrail.expert
FB: www.facebook.com/EllieBorden
Twitter: https://twitter.com/EllieBorden

### Sexy Beast Lingerie

Web:www.sexybeastlingerie.com
FB: www.facebook.com/SexyBeastBoutique
Twitter: https://twitter.com/LingeriePalace

### PowerCircle

Web: www.powercircleacademy.com FB:
www.facebook.com/POWERCIRCLEACADEMY
Twitter: https://twitter.com/PowerCircleAcad

### Title:
My Journey to Wholeness

### Subtitle:
I have a need to soar to feel full in my core

### Author:
Ellie Borden

# 12

## BLAZING THE TRAIL

### Trinidadian Culinarian Cops The Cover Of Toastmasters Magazine

- BY SHELLY-ANN WILLIAMS, OWNER AND EXECUTIVE CHEF
OF FIREWOOD FOOD STOP.

Cool, calm and candid are the words commonly used to describe Shelly-Ann Lovell-Willams, a Trinidadian Toastmaster who has moved from being a timid procrastinator to becoming a template of success for women in Trinidad and Tobago and the Caribbean.

In her two and a half years of being a Toastmaster, Shelly-Ann rose from presenting short speeches to an audience of 20, to showcasing her leadership skills on the cover of an international magazine.

So how does an easy-going Trinidadian chef end up being featured on the front cover ofan 80 year old magazine? Well, here's how she did it!

Shelly-Ann first heard of Toastmasters International in 2011 when she was hired to do photography for an event hosted at a hotel in Trinidad. When she first heard the name Toastmasters, she immediately thought this was an international alcoholic beverage company that was launching in her country by hostng a tasting session for locals. She gushed at the thought of being in the presence of wine conossieurs, not to mention the multiple wine and spirit tasting for the evening.

After her entrance at the venue, she noticed that there were no alcoholic beverages on-site and thought that since it was such a large company, the tasting was probably going to be held in a separate room. What she couldn't understatd was the connection to the dozens of public speakers at the event who constantly made mention of communication and leadership skills. "This must be a really elite association that marries communication skills with alcohol tasting", she thought.

Though she anticipated getting to the tasting session after the meeting, she was however impressed by the presentation skills of all speakers and became interested in their speaking abilities.

She was particularly intrigued by a session that was coined, *Table Topics*, which was the art of impromptu speaking through the answering of random questions. This she saw as a challenge she would like to attempt. Questions were based on Trinidad folklore and she realized that she had the capability to answer most without faltering. Instead of tasting of delicious wines, beers and spirits that evening, Shelly-Ann left the event with a taste for more of Toastmasters and a flavour for improving her speaking skills.

One year later she decided to satisfy that hunger by visiting a Toastmasters club in Arima, Trinidad and there she fell in love again, with Table Topics. This time she was afforded the opportunity to participate and enjoyed the meeting immensely. The following month she joined the Nepuyo Toastmasters club and began her journey to speaking excellence.

Four months later she was asked to be nominated as the Vice President Public Relations of the club by her mentors at the next club elections. She was hesitant at first, considering that she was new to the organization and hadn't known much of the requirements of being on the Executive. She eventually obliged and was voted into the position in June, 2013.

Shelly-Ann immediately began reseaching and reading about the organization in order to maximize her potential as a club leader. This feat helped her in creating a Public Relations plan for her club and spreading the good news of Toastmasters to fellow Trinidadians.

Her next exploit was entering the Humorous Speech competition at club level. Since she was at Project five – Your Body Speaks, in the Competent Communicator manual, she performed a hilarious speech about a character named Sister Shugs who was known for her charismatic behaviour in the streets. This presentation won her first place in he competition, her first contest achievement even before she celebrated her first anniversary as a member. She then won the Area and National Competition within the next month and represented her country at the District 81 (Caribbean) Humorous Speech competition Puerto Rico in 2013. Although she did not place in that competition, she made a firm decision to compete again the following year, where she again represented Trinidad and Tobago at the Caribbean contest and walked away with the first prize for Humorous Speech in St Lucia in 2014.

Shelly-Ann's avid love for Toastmasters led to her nickname, "no problem Shelly", as she found it difficult to turn down a challenge without at least making an attempt. This was the case when she was challenged by the President of the Student Guild of a local university, Cipriani College of Labour and Cooperative Studies, to be the master of ceremonies for a three day retreat. Shelly-Ann was the Public Relations representative on the Guild and had settled herself to relax and enjoy the weekend retreat with fellow members.

The President approached her ten minutes before the start of the retreat and said, "Can you be the master of ceremonies for the entire event?" Only being a toastmaster for six months, Shelly-Ann was poised to prove that she could do the job. She asked for a 20 minute dely and proceeded to create biographies for the three facilitators by conducting short five minute interviews with them. She then did a quick online research on the theme of the event, "Chartering the Course for good Student Governance"and the show began.

Her calm confident character made a strong statement as she likened the retreat to a ship on its course to success and describing the facilitators as several types of seamen as she read their biographies.

The Director of the College was so impressed with her presentation that he commended her on what the thought was her daily job. He was astonished to find out that her attribution to such a great performance was the fact that she was a Toastmaster. He later understood that Toastmasters International was a non-profit organization in 126 countries with a membership of 313,000 worldwide and the world leader in communication and leadership development.

This was the beginning of the Cips Power Achivers Toastmasters, the club she started at the College in November, 2013 where she served as Vice President – Education.

The club had a slow start due to several challenges in the beginning, however, that was not enough to quench the leadership fire within her. She continued to train the few interested students in the roles and responsibilities of a Toastmaster and provide support for the fearful and shy guests who visited the club. In addition, she received support from her home club and mentors and the club eventually became chartered in March, 2015, notwithstanding, they attained the level of Distinguished Club within the first two months of chatering.

Shelly-Ann's hardworking nature has been applauded both within Toastmasters and in the corporate world. Due to her bubbly personality and ability to make others laugh, she was invited to be the host of an annual concert held by the Trinidad and Tobago Steel and Brass Symphonic Orchestra in July, 2013. Being the mother of two of the members of the band, Jassiem and Nyah, she was more than delighted to again use her Toastmastering skills. The event showcased young musicians from ages seven to eighteen playing various instruments including steelpan, flute, clarinet, trombone, saxophone and trumpet. She spent weeks preparing for the occasion, doing research on the band, music in Trinidad and Tobago and history of the songs being performed. She even developed games for audience participation.

The show was a smashing success, as several of the patrons praised her for keeping the audience engaged and jovial. After her first show, she was accoladed by the executive of the band and retained as the master of ceremonies for all four shows held annually.

This opened other speaking engagements for Shelly-Ann as she was invited to host another large scaled show themed Red Runway, which featured dozens of local fashion designers and over 200 fashion models in a two day event. She was again retained as the annual host of this show.

Shelly-Ann has also been the host of an online cooking series with a local television company and has hosted carnival band launches, beauty pageants, fund raisers, sport events and corporate events.

In October,2013, an Australian Tostmaster sent an email to Toastmasters around the world in search of talented artists to be featured in his book, *101 Toastmasters Around the World.* The book was set to showcase the artistic talent of Toastmasters globally and  Shelly-Ann immediately indicated her interest and began collating content for the feature.

Over the next few months, she worked tirelessly on getting the final story together  then eagerly awaited publication in 2014.  The book was launched  later that year and showcased ShellyAnn's life as a photographer. At that time, she owned Shellyfossick Studio, a local based video and photography business that recorded still photographs, corporate photography and video recording for weddings, events and also government and private institutions.  The recognition received from the book boosted Shelly-Ann's confidence in her daily endeavours, which also included working on her Toastmasters education awards.

This confidence was acknowledged by a church in her community, that invited her to conduct a dream building workshop for women.  The workshop was attended by 30 women ranging from teenagers to senior citizens and touched on the six steps of goal setting. Women were assisted with  choosing an area  in their lives, where they wanted to achieve some type of success and practically setting the goals to achieve them.  Areas included improvement of education, weight loss, overcoming fears and starting businesses.  Part of the session included writing down all challenges in getting to the ultimate goal and setting timelines for achieving them. They were then given the following six months to begin executing their plans and a review was scheduled after expiration of the time. The results of the workshop was phenomenal, as several of the women admitted that they never thought of making a step by step plan to achieveing goals or actually overcoming the fear of failure which caused the initial procrastination.

Shelly-Ann's journey became more exciting as she began the Advanced level of the Toastmasters communication and leadership programmes. With several more projects to present, she always took pleasure in adding a bit of humour in her deliveries.  She became noted for her alluring presentations as she  cleverly softened strong messages with a hint of humour.  This was apparent in her message entitled, *Dont Judge a Book by its Cover,* which dramatized a woman accusing her partner of being unfaithful, when he was caught in the presence of another woman who ultimately turned out to be his cousin.

Her affinity to keeping her audience engaged was evident when she teamed up with Trinidadian author Lyndon Baptiste for a book launch of *Jewels of the Caribbean* in October, 2014. The book was a collection of short stories by some of the finest emerging Caribbean writers and focused on life in the West Indies with comical situations and conclusions. Minutes before the performance, Shelly-Ann tripped and fell down a staircase and sprained her right ankle,however this was never a deterrant to her spirit. She performed, *Sweet Hand*, the first story in the book, which was a tale of jealousy between two female vendors of an elementary school. Her dramatization created a raucous frenzy as the audience immensely enjoyed the presentation. Even the author of the story was surprised at the performance, since the two had never met or communicated with each other before that day. "Shelly-Ann captured the character of Tantie Mona, exactly as I created her and I look forward to working with her again in the future", said the author.

In January, 2015, Shelly-Ann received a message from a foreignToastmaster friend asking her interest in participating in an article for the Toastmaster magazine. The article focused on international chefs and leadership in the kitchen with attention given to how chefs interact with their protegés as they impart leadership skills for further development. The topic was an intimate one for Shelly-Ann as she had been in the culinary industry for over 20 years and was accustomed to training young people in the areas of food preparation, baking and pastry arts, sugar artistry and food service. Without hesitation, she agreed and was contacted by an Editor, later that week. This was followed by a telephone interview by the writer of the story and contact with proof readers.

Her next stop was a photo shoot which included guidelines for a possible front cover photo. Shelly-Ann was intrigued by the thought of being on the cover of a magazine that distributes to over 300,000 members worldwide butconsidered that her chances of this actually happening, was slim since she had only been a Toastmaster for two years and she had never seen any Toastmaster featured on the cover. The shoot was done at her restaurant, Firewood Food Stop with her nephew and Line Cook, Shaquel Lovell. The evening was a blast as customers enjoyed some fun with the chef and were even lucky enough to walk away with some recipe tips!

After the captioned photos were submitted to Toastmasters International, there was the one month wait for the release of the May issue which seemed like almost a year as she eagerly awaited the viewing.

One afternoon in early May, as she was in her home office, she heard the creaking of the mail box as her mom was retrieving mail. "There's your mom!", were the words uttered to her children who were playing in the garage. Shelly-Ann knew that it could only mean that she was on the front cover of the magazine. Her shriek was heard metres away as she pranced all over the office with her kids, pleasantly surprised to see herself on the cover of the magazine she had enjoyed reading for the past two years. Within the next week she received numerous calls and contact from Toastmasters all over the Caribbean who were elated to see a fellow Toastmaster on their favourite magazine. In the following weeks she enjoyed receiving congratulations from internationally recognized World Champion Speakers, District Directors, international speakers and Toastmasters from across the globe.

One of the local daily newpapers in Trinidad even granted her a feature story in thier woman magazine and several more speaking engagements opened up due to her international recognition.

Shelly-Ann's passion for helping others overcome their fear of public speaking has helped many of her peers face their weaknesses. She now has her heart set on conducting Youth Leadership Programmes for the young adults in her community. She plans to help them develop the art of public speaking, communication skills and leadership through the Toastmasters programme. In addition, she also looks forward to hosting dream building workshops to assist individuals in creating practical plans towards achieving their dreams.

Currently she is at the level of Advanced Communicator Gold and Advanced Leadership Silver in the Toastmasters Educational Programme and will be receiving her Triple Crown award in October, 2015 for achieving three education awards in one year.

Although she has been actively promoting the Toastmasters brand in her country, she attributes her achievements to the support of her family. Her parents Peter and Idris and only sibling, Sean, have been a pillar of strength to her in her educational expedition.

Her life-partner, Stephen, joined Toastmasters in 2013, after seeing her perform at a National Humorous contest and remains her number one fan and source of inspiration. They both enjoy empowering students and guests at thier club and motivating each other as they pursue their speaking aspirations.

Of course, her three beautiful gems, Jassiem, 11; Nyah, 9 and Jahiem, 6, eagerly await their future opportunity to become members of Toastmasters. In the meantime, the three accomplished musicians practice their speaking skills under the guidance of their enthusiastic mom.

Shelly-Ann believies in the words of United States statesman Colin Powel, "A dream doesn't become reality through magic, it takes sweat, determination and hard work." A quote she has seen operative in her life throughout the years and will continue to cultivate in anyone she encounters.

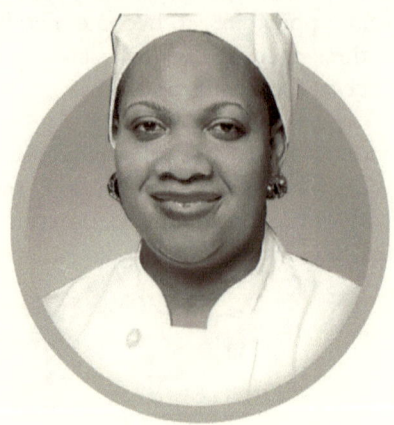

**Shelly-Ann Lovell-Williams**

Shelly-Ann Lovell-Williams has been a Toastmaster for two and a half years and attributes her success to the communication and leadership skills developed through the Toastmasters Educational Programme. The mother of three enjoys empowering others to reach for their goals and overcome their fear of public speaking.

Some of her speaking successes include winning the District 81 (Caribbean) Toastmasters Humorous Speaking contest in October, 2014, two-time National Humorous Speaker in 2013 and 2014; host of several local events; motivational speaker and mentor.

In 2013 she founded the Cips Power Achievers Toastmasters Club at the Cipriani College of Labour and Cooperative Studies and is also a member of Nepuyo Toastmasters, Trinidad.

Shelly-Ann firmly believes that goals can be achieved through persistence and hard work, both of which will help you realize your ultimate dreams.

# 13

## A HEALER'S JOURNEY

**The road to finding the ever evolving upward spiral of my heart centered existence.**

- BY DR. DEBBIE NOVICK, A LEADING EXPERT ON HASHIMOTO'S THYROIDITIS.

It all began when I was born 55 years ago in Mexico City to American parents.

I was fortunate to be raised in luxury, and next door to me, on the other side of the wall of my home (mansion really), lived a family in a tin and cardboard shack. At the age of 8 years old, I became painfully aware that I could not reconcile this duality without making a concerted effort to contribute in some way, and change the world I was experiencing. My burning desire to fill my life purpose with finding a way to rectify this enormous disparity of existence was ignited by this awareness.

In addition, my younger sister was born with severe dyslexia and hyperactivity. In those days, the 1960's, there was no understanding or recognition of these disabilities. Consequently, my sister suffered innumerable physical and psychological injury until the age of 11. After watching her suffer and struggle, at the age of 16 or 17, I decided I would become a special education teacher. At the time, I was convinced this was my life's purpose.

So I pursued this goal and became a special education teacher by moving to the United States when I was nearly 18 years old and graduating with a BA in Psychology and Regular and Special Education credentials at age of 23.

After spending 6 years as a special education teacher, I became aware that the institution that provided me a place to pour my life's mission into was not in alignment with my vision of the legacy I wished to leave behind. In this environment, with this vocation, I would not be able to make a difference.

So after pondering on what career would be next in serving my purposes, because of the many times I had been saved as a patient, I was led to consider becoming a chiropractor and alternative medicine practitioner.

I knew that this would make my life's purpose and passion a much more powerful and impactful statement. Having the opportunity to heal the world one person at a time, is a much more meaningful legacy to leave behind.

At the age of 31, I went back to school to gather the necessary prerequisites, began chiropractic school at the age of 33, learning that I was pregnant two weeks before my studies began at Life West Chiropractic College. I happened to be living 75 miles away from the college and had to commute 5 days a week. As I look back at that time in my life, I am amazed at the determination and commitment I had to accomplish my mission. It took a super human effort to move through the challenges of pregnancy while immersing myself in a highly demanding curriculum. I was determined to reach my goal, and after 3.5 years, I graduated valedictorian of my class and began my new career.

In my 19 years in practice I was fortunate to be exposed to and sought training from many talented people. Constantly seeking to learn more, I continued to attend postgraduate courses that would add strategic and innovative tools to my practice. My intention was to give the highest quality care as I was consumed with a commitment to provide excellence.

I endured the ravages of the stress of school, starting a practice, and letting go of my devastatingly dysfunctional marriage, subsequently facing the challenging task of raising my emotionally challenged son, as a single working mother. In addition, once I began practicing, I was faced with the risks of the repetitive motion daily activities of my work. I was injured and nearly disabled on several occasions. I refused to succumb; my desire for learning, led me to natural and alternative solutions to all my injuries and illnesses along the way. I have always had a strong intuitive and keenly observant mind, which has served me well. Gratefully, thanks to my milieu, I over came the possibility of having to retire and re-invent myself with each disabling physical challenge.

Despite my good fortune, after 2 decades of unending stress, as I was approaching menopause, and heading for a big health challenge slowly but surely. Even though intellectually I was aware that stress does kill, I was unconsciously, painfully, walking around allowing the deleterious effects to gradually break down my body, mind, and spirit's wellness. Driving myself to always push through, work endlessly; accomplish goals, focusing on doing more, being more for others, and leaving myself on the back burner. This took my DIS-EASE train to a supersonic speed journey towards a health-devastating destination.

I want to share with you the journey I took from a state of illness and distress to glorious health and vitality. As well as, delineate how that changed the focus of my practice and the women I became passionate about serving and supporting.

Here's the story of how I came to be here today and why I care so much about what I am called to do. I have been in practice for 19 years dedicating myself to serving hundreds of patients. I stand here before you in better health and having more vitality than I have since I was in high school. I own my own business, am single and enjoy my life.

I have had the luxury and freedom to travel internationally, visiting places like Nepal, New Zealand, England, and Thailand, which has given me a much broader perspective in understanding the diversity of health challenges on the planet, as well as my own. The lifestyle and economic standard of living play important roles in the quality of health and kinds of medicine used. This has driven me to be even more passionate about helping my patients, given the quality of care I can provide them.

But things were not always this way.... In April of 2012, I felt out of control with my life. I was struggling with insomnia, exhausted all the time 24/7 hot flashes for 6 weeks (I was using all that I knew could help yet nothing was changing), i gained 20-30 pounds off and on during that time... this seemed to all be the result of 15 years of struggling with 3 major stressful experiences; completing graduate school while pregnant, going through a rough divorce, and then hitting menopause.

I was so desperate, I was guided in the right direction to get blood tests and an advisor to help me see what was at the root cause of it all.

After speaking with my friend and functional medicine mentor Datis Kharrazian D.C., etc., who looked at my lab test results and said to me, "Debbie, you have 5 years." When I heard this, I felt like it was life or death if I did not do something now!

Being told I had 5 years to live, I realized the trouble I was in and committed to learning the answers to what was killing my body. I hate to imagine had I waited any longer to seek support!

I realized I had a choice, I could continue on this out of control journey, or I could chose to taking matters into my own hands and make the necessary dietary and lifestyle choices that would result in life and vitality.

I immediately took it upon myself to embark on my own healing journey by implementing an anti-inflammatory diet, supplements, increased my fitness activities, and integrated stress reducing strategies and exercises.

I sought professional support in other areas of expertise. Even though I was, and am a skilled expert, there were some things I was missing. I asked Datis (remind that he is my mentor) as well as other practitioners at seminars I attended, who had embarked on similar journeys, how they were coping and finding ways to succeed.

Gradually I became stronger and learned to balance my busy stressful life with making healthy food, exercise, rest, and fun a priority, and finding ways to stay accountable by getting support around me.

I always feel better when I get to share things with other professionals I respect and trust. Especially those I can say anything to, and they listen and support me through it, offering valuable perspectives and ideas.

It was challenging at first to let go of the foods I loved, yet I knew there could be nutritious and delicious ways to get my health back so I actually ended up creating new recipes that have been turned into a cookbook. My book will be out in bookstores July 2015.

This journey inspired me to serve, and here I am today, blessed to be able to share it. So after this experience of feeling so out of control and getting back in control. I now know the path of taming the out of control health challenges. I have been there myself, and am so passionate about helping my patients go from feeling out of control to taming Hashimoto's.
.

My intention is that my patients tame Hashimoto's and other chronic conditions, so they can feel, energized, and in control again, more specifically, that they will have practical tips and strategies to empower them for life to overcome any health challenges and bring back a JOY for life.

Now as I go into my 20th year in practice, I am not only focused on serving women with Hashimoto's, I am also driven to create a revolution in the health care system of the world. One in which each and every person will know how to stay healthy and vital throughout their lives.

Rather than focusing on DIS-EASE, diagnosis, and symptom relief, focusing on lifestyle and dietary practices that keep the body/mind healthy, vibrant, and active until we decide to leave our physical form.

The challenges of the modern world pose many obstacles to achieving optimal health. The erosion of nutrients in the organic food that is shipped to grocery stores, GMO's, packaged foods, sugar, drugs (legal or not), poor air quality, 1000's of toxic chemicals, over used farmland, carbon dioxide emissions, heavy metals, infections, emotional and physical stress, sedentary lifestyles, electro pollution; cell phones, wires overhead, microwaves, home phones, computers. The list is long and creates an enormous challenge to our fragile yet miraculous and finely tuned body.

It is no wonder there are so many people suffering from degenerative diseases and the numbers are growing, due to the current model of modern medicine.

People are being prescribed drugs that only mask the problems created by modern living, they keep people sold on the idea that they need another magic pill to deal with symptoms created by the first drug, and so on, and so on. It's time to find another solution.

So how on earth does one keep this body/mind finely humming?

The key is to look to nature and know that the bounty of what this amazing planet we live in offers is infinite. I believe that everything has a purpose and all living and non-living things on earth have life-giving properties to the processes that keep the body/mind supported and able to adapt to the many challenges we face today.

The other parts of maintaining a body/mind healthy entail putting attention to having positive and intimate relationships with an extended family and surrounding community. One in which each child born has a loving caring group of people that contributes to their development.

Without touch, the immune system and brain do not develop to their full potential. Finding ways to connect with others is vital to health.

Just like the body requires that its nervous system, immune system, and endocrine system (glands; adrenal, pancreas, liver, thyroid, pituitary, etc) work together in an interlocking network of connections and feedback loops that are inseparable.

As they say "no man lives on an island." The body/mind cannot be put into boxes and treated as tough each part is a separate entity. The connections are everywhere and everything affects everything else.

The triad of health is to balance the emotional, chemical, and physical states of the body. There is an incredible plethora of modalities and tools today that address this triad. My legacy will be to create a source of information. One that will provide a platform that anyone with health challenges, can take a journey to discover exactly what magic combination of modalities, tools, or people, will restore them to full health and wellness.

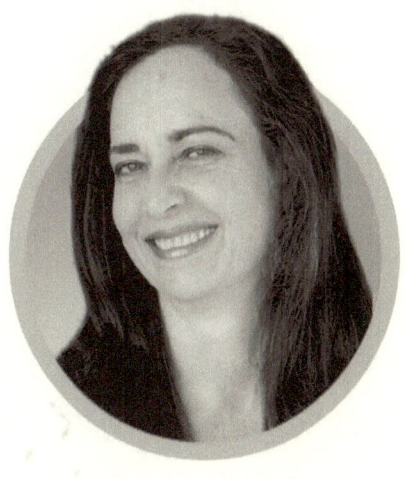

**Dr. Debbie Novick, DC**

Debbie Novick, D.C., a leading expert on Hashimoto's Thyroiditis, practices at the renowned Novick Integrated Medicine in Encinitas, CA. Educated and trained at Life Chiropractic College West in Hayward, CA, Dr. Debbie has continued her postgraduate studies in functional and integrative medicine, specializing in women's health care and nutrition. She uses a variety of natural health care practices such as N.E.T. chiropractic care for mental-emotional clearing, Bach flower remedies, and homeopathic remedies to restore health and balance to her patients. Known as the "Go-to Doctor" for Hashimoto's, Dr. Debbie works in concert with other MD's and Gynecologists who refer their patients to her for more specialized autoimmune support.

**Website: http://www.drdebnov.com**

# 14

# HOW TO BUILD AN AUTHORITY BLOG

## - BY VINIL RAMDEV, ENTREPRENEUR, EDITOR AND MARKETER.

I started doing business on the internet way back in 2004. Social media wasn't such a big rage at the time. Social media sites like friendster and Hi5 were considered pretty much trivial to make any sort of impact in the business world. Blogs were still around at the time, and it was fairly inexpensive to start blogging.

In 2006, I was running a retail pharmacy business in India and I was also taking some online classes at the Trump University (now called Trump Entrepreneur Initiative). I wasn't sure why I started blogging, I didn't know the reason, it just appealed to me and I started writing blog posts. I was writing about my business and pretty much everything under the sun. I didn't even have a domain of my own, I just started blogging by signing up with blogger.com, which was a free platform. At the time I would write about one blog post a month.

After several years I started a very successful blog in the start-up niche, which I eventually sold as I wanted to move on to other niches. The reason for me to start a business blog was primarily to sell my consulting services. At the time, I had made a transition into business consulting and I was looking to offer my services to potential clients. One of the best ways to sell my services was to start a blog and position myself as a knowledgeable person.

I DO NOT believe that everything in this chapter is the gospel of blogging. It is NOT. Feel free to disagree, and experiment as you wish. Each of the methods I have listed are merely suggestions. Some of the methods might work for you and some may not. If it resonates with you, go ahead and try them, if it does not work for you then discard them.

### What is an authority blog?

An authority blog is a blog that positions you as a knowledgeable person in your field. It sets you up as the go-to person for a particular topic.

### Why should you build an authority blog?

Anybody who is trying to sell his products or services should consider blogging.

An authority blog,
Builds your reputation
Gives you a voice
Gives your potential customers a sample of what you have to offer

### What makes a blog stand out from the crowd?

There are basically just three things that make a blog stand out from the crowd.
Good Design
Great Content
Personal connection with the blogger

### What makes great content?

The purpose of any content is to inform, educate, entertain, or sell a product or service. When someone visits your blog, he is looking for a solution to one of his problems, or is merely looking to entertain himself. Good blogs try to solve their reader's problems.

## Blog Design

I, personally, like blog designs that are simple and have a lot of white space. The trend in blog design is towards simple, easy to navigate designs. Be careful about placing Google ads in every corner of your blog. It is very tempting to place ads everywhere but resist the temptation and use ads sparingly.

## Choosing a blog topic

This is a very common question for most people starting off in blogging. I tell people to write about something they are doing on a day-to-day basis. When you are doing something on a day-to-day basis, it is very easy to come up with article ideas, and topics to write about. You could write about your day job, or a hobby you are passionate about. For example, if you are a web designer, write about web designing. If you are a cook, write about cooking. Most people think they are not experts at anything, but the fact is that most people are experts at something or the other. Just observe how you spend your time, and you'll find a topic to blog about.

## The simple ways...

## Identify your reasons for blogging

When I started a business blog, my reason for blogging was to sell my consulting services. My blog helped me position myself as a knowledgeable person in my niche and it also gave my prospects an indication of my business acumen.

There are several other reasons to start a blog. One of the reasons could be that you want your voice to be heard and blogging could be a great way to be heard.

Another reason could be to make money from your blogs. During the initial stages, it may be really hard to make money from your blog because you barely have any traffic, but as you build traffic, there are ways you could make money from blogging.

Networking can be another reason to start blogging. There are possibilities to meet several people online through blogging. Whatever your reasons, it helps to know why you want to blog. If you are not sure why you want to blog, you could still get started blogging and identify your reasons along the way.

### Find a niche

This is a very clichéd statement in the blogging world. But it makes a lot of sense. Initially you may wander around and write about a variety of topics ranging from football to marketing to dating but eventually it is very likely that you could burn out.

The reason you should find a profitable niche and stick to it is because people see you as the go-to person on that topic and people want to talk to experts and not always generalists when they are looking at things like "how to finance a business" or "how to startup a business." You may want to focus on specific skill sets and be the best at it rather than be a jack of all trades and a master of none.

Most people know this but they still try a lot of different things. I am one of them. I have broken this rule several times. I have tried a lot of businesses in my life and the reason for that, is, I did not find a profitable business in my first attempt. But yes, eventually I do understand that I need to find a niche and be the best at it.

Coming back to blogging, it makes sense to choose a niche because it will make your job a lot easier. Sometime niches can be really broad, so it is important you find the right balance. For example, if you are an event planner and you are focused on every event category from weddings to trade shows to fashion shows, you have to now spread your wings among several different markets. Weddings is a different market, fashion shows are a different market, trade shows are a whole different market altogether. Promoting yourself in several different markets is really difficult because your resources are going to be too spread out to make any real impact.

### Blog Frequently

Nothing can kill a blog faster than infrequent blogging. You cannot just blog once in three months or once in six months or even once a month. You need to blog at least once a week. I know people who have a full time job, but they still blog every day.

It might initially be difficult for you to blog everyday because you have never done it before. If you start doing it, it's going to get easier and easier every day. It's like building muscle.

Search engines also rank websites higher when they are being updated frequently.

### Provide great content

It goes without saying that GREAT CONTENT is what makes blogs stand out. Every blog is trying to differentiate itself from the other with it's content. Some blogs consist of predominately "How-to" type articles, others have a more personal tone with reality based articles, while there are others that are a combination of both.

Whatever format of articles you'd like to adopt for your blog, try to find your own voice, be authentic, and be yourself..

### Keep in touch with your blog readers

Once you are blogging frequently and people start frequenting your blog, you must have some way of staying in touch with your readers. Not collecting information about your blog readers is like going to a business conference, talking to people and just walking away without exchanging business cards.

One way to keep in touch with your blog readers is a mailing list. Your blog should have some sort of form to collect email addresses. It is quite easy to create an automated mailing list. Softwares like aweber.com, constantcontact.com help you collect email addresses of your blog readers. Remember, your blog readers have to fill up a form on your website to be added into your mailing list. Not all your readers would want to sign up on your mailing list, but even if 5% of your blog readers sign up, it's still better than nothing.

A lot of people might be apprehensive to sign up for your mailing list because people get so much of spam every day. What you do is, give them an incentive to sign up for your mailing list. The incentive could be a discount coupon, it could be a report, or even an eBook.

If you would like to know more about setting up a mailing list for your website, you can visit aweber.com, constantcontact.com or mailchimp.com and learn more about setting up a mailing list for your blog.

Another way of staying in touch with your blog readers is a Facebook page, Twitter, LinkedIn or many of the several online social networks.

Every time you write a blog post, update your social networks with that blog entry and people could come back and take a look at your blog post if the headline interests them.

### Guest post on other people's blogs

Guest posting is nothing but writing an article on other people's blogs. The advantage with guest posting is that you are exposed to a whole new audience. It is also possible to get leads and improve traffic to your blog from each of your guest posts. Guest posting is also a great opportunity for you to improve your reputation.

A prospective client who wanted to hire me did a Google search about me and he found several pages of information about me. I was everywhere. This enhanced my reputation and I got the gig. So, even if you don't get traffic to your blog (which rarely happens unless you choose a blog host with no traffic at all), the worst case scenario of guest posting is that it will improve your reputation.

Another advantage with guest blogging is that it builds your SEO. When you guest post, blog owners let you leave a link at the end of your article. Backlinks help build the SEO ranking of your own blog.

But please be careful when choosing places to guest post. Choose websites that look professional and have at least some sort of traffic.

It is not very difficult to get guest posting opportunities. You can find guest posting opportunities on websites like bloggerlinkup.com or myblogguest.com. Once you sign up on these websites, they email you a list of bloggers who are looking for guest posts.

Consequently, get other experts to guest post on your blog. Once your blog develops a good page rank and has a good readership base, it will become attractive for other people to guest post on your blog.

### How **<u>NOT</u>** to make a guest post offer?

Several people send me guest posts to put up on my blog. A big majority of the guest posts get rejected. The reason many of these guest posts get rejected is because bloggers don't present themselves very well.

Some of the most common mistakes include:

*Not introducing themselves* – Lot of people just send me a blog post without telling me who they are or what topic they plan on presenting. I like people who send me a list of topics with a brief description of each topic. This gives me an option to choose a topic most suitable for me.

*Sending frivolous emails* like "do you accept guest posts" or "I can guest blog for you" – Remember, A-list bloggers usually get so many emails that you don't want to waste their time sending frivolous emails like "do you accept guest posts?" I had someone send me a blog post offer that read "I will blog for you. Just say the word. Etc etc.." This is just not the way to approach someone. In the next few paragraphs, I will show you exactly how to make an offer.

*Following up too soon* – Sometimes people send an email and follow-up within 6 to 8 hours with another email – did you get my message? Following-up within 12 hrs? Gimme a break. If you don't get a reply back, just let it go and offer your blog post to another blog. If you really want to follow-up, follow-up after 2 weeks, never before that.

*Writing extremely formal and stiff emails* – Business has changed over the years, formal and stiff emails don't work. Be professional but don't write emails that are a template from the 1970s book of business letters.

*Getting too personal and emotional* – Just don't rant and throw tantrums if you don't get a reply. You need to remember that the blog owner has no obligation to publish your guest post. So just because you've put in the effort to write the guest post does not mean it gives you a right to be published. There are several reasons blog owners don't reply – like – not enough time to review guest posts, more emails than they can handle, sometimes the guest post is not a fit with their blog, etc.

*Deceptive subject lines* – This is another big turn-off. Your subject line should never be deceptive. If you are writing to a blog owner about a blog post offer, make sure you mention it in the subject line.

*Being Arrogant and selling a grandiose plan* – Sometimes blog owners get an email that says, "I am offering the following articles on a first come first serve basis. You are the lucky one who this email is going to. Reply soon or this offer will not exist." Unless you are Richard Branson or Bill Gates, this is a very naïve way to pitch your services.

### How to make a Guest Post Offer?

Now, coming to *how to do it right...*

When you are writing an email to make a guest post offer, it is important you do it right, and do it professionally.

Step 1: Introduce yourself.

Your introduction should be brief and don't make it more than 2 or 3 lines at the most. It could be something like "I am John Smith – the founder of simpleblogs.com, a blog about simplicity."

Step 2: Mention the reason for the email.

Your reason could go like, "I am writing to see if I could be a guest poster on your website – websitename.com"

Step 3: Write a list of topics you would like to blog about.

Your blog topics should include a headline and a brief description of the article you propose to write.

For example: "*I plan to write a guest post on the following topics:*

*10 places to meet your soul mate*

*This topic introduces people to unique and little known places where girls and guys can hang out to meet their soul mate. My sources for this article include various people who have found their soul mates in unconventional places.....*"

Step 4: Have an appropriate subject line

As mentioned in the previous pages, do not write a deceptive subject line. I like to have a subject line like "Guest Post for XYZ blog." This ensures the blog owner that you are sending an email specifically to him and not sending a bulk email. You may also want to include one of your article headlines in the subject line to catch the blog owner's attention.

Step 5: Send a Thank You note

This is something so many guest posters forget or don't bother doing. Guest posting is an opportunity to build a relationship with other bloggers. Although this does not seem very important, it is a crucial part of the guest blogging experience. Once your guest post is published, don't forget to send a *thank you* email, it's just courtesy.

### How I choose which blogs to guest post on?

Obviously you may not want to guest post on each and every blog that gives you an opportunity. You may want to be selective, because everytime you guest post on someone else's blog, you are giving up time that could be used to build your own blog.

Find below, how I choose the blogs to guest post on.

#1 I like to guest post on blogs where I frequently read articles, or at least like their content.

#2 The blog should be professional looking. I don't like to guest post on blogs that are not professional looking. If the blog owner has not taken the time to build a professional looking blog then that's not a blog I want to consider guest blogging on.

#3 The blog should be updated frequently. If the last post on that blog was 3 months ago, that to me is lack of commitment.

#4 The blog should have a high alexa ranking. I like to post on blogs with an alexa ranking above 250,000. If a blog is ranked way below 250,000, that does NOT mean it is a deal breaker. I would still look at other factors before making my decision.

#5 The blog should have a clean layout. If there are more Google ads than there are articles, then that's not a blog I would like to guest post on.

#6 Finally, if I have a great feeling about the blog. And the blog owner has interacted with me honestly with humility, passion, enthusiasm, and is willing to go to great lengths to have me guest post on his blog, I might just oversee all the above factors.

## Comment on other people's blogs

Commenting on other people's blog is something I've seen work. I discovered this when I started commenting on social media examiner, when I checked my Google analytics I saw several clicks coming from social media examiner and all this was because of commenting. But be very careful. Do not spam. Make a well-thought through comment. It is very tempting to spam, but resist the temptation to spam and make a comment with a purpose of connecting with someone rather than trying to sell something.

You also don't have to put your website link in the comments box because what happens on many of these blogs is that you can enter a website, an email address and your name. Your email won't be visible of course but your name will be a hyperlink. So when people click on your name, they are directed to your blog. I have never left my website address ever in any of my comments but somehow people reply to my comment and the discussion starts. Comment with an objective to start a conversation with somebody rather than trying to get a click to your blog.

### Yahoo Answers

I still get several clicks to my blog from Yahoo Answers even though I stopped answering questions on Yahoo Answers a long time ago. If you go to answers.yahoo.com, you will see several questions for which people are seeking answers. You may choose to answer as many questions as you like, and in the end of the thread there is a box called source(s) – you can leave your website url as the source which will help you get some clicks to your blog.

Another advantage with Yahoo Answers is that it is a great source for article ideas. You can generate article ideas from the questions people want answered.

### Give out information that helps your readers

One of the reasons people visit blogs is to get information about events happening in their neighborhood. For example, on my blog I put out information about business plan competitions. This was a benefit for my readers who are mostly entrepreneurs and business owners. If your blog is constantly putting up information that benefits your readers, this gives your readers reasons to come back and visit your blog. The question you need to constantly keep asking yourself is "how can I benefit my readers?"

## Making money from your blog - 4 income streams

A lot of people want to know how they can make money from their blog. Not all income streams maybe applicable to your blog but some of them might apply to your blog.

### Income Stream #1 - Advertising

This is the most common way of monetizing your blog.

It is very simple to sign up for a Google adsense account at http://www.google.com/adsense or several other ad networks like adbrite, federated media, infolinks, etc. You could also sell ads directly to businesses, which is a little bit more difficult and time consuming for new blogs. A lot of blog owners just prefer a self-serviced ad network where they don't have to expend any time on selling ads.

### Income Stream #2 – Subscriptions

If you don't want to give away your content for FREE, you can have subscribers pay for your content. There are several wordpress plugins like wishlist that can convert a wordpress blog into a subscription based website.

### Income Stream #3 – Ebooks and Webinars

Another way for blogs to make money is by selling ebooks and webinars. Some bloggers have had enormous success by converting their blog posts into ebooks. This is another opportunity to generate income and monetize your blog.

### Income Stream #4 – Commission from Affiliate Sales

If you don't have your own products, you can recommend other people's products and make money from it. When you sign up as an affiliate, you are given a link with an affiliate id that you post on your website, whenever someone clicks on the link and buys a product you get a referral commission. It is also called CPA or cost per action. It is a good idea to always choose affiliate products that you like, or use.

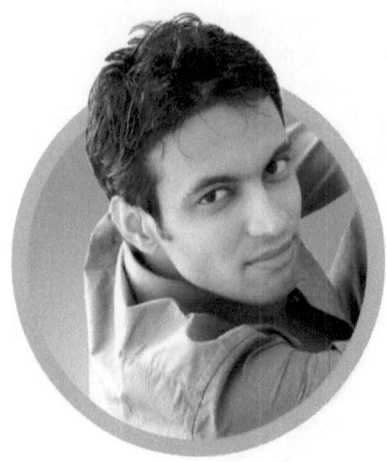

### Vinil Ramdev

Vinil Ramdev, entrepreneur, editor, marketer, was born in Bangalore, India, attended college at Florida Atlantic University in Boca Raton, Florida in the United States of America where he graduated with a Bachelors degree in Marketing in 2004. Since then, Vinil has been involved in starting and growing several businesses predominantly in retail, marketing, media, advertising and on the internet. His skill for seeing the big picture, and identifying trends and patterns have made him a sort-after consultant for companies who want to grow their business and make their products more discoverable.

Vinil is also the Managing Editor of a nationally circulated print magazine in India. He participated in NDTV's hot debate "SMEs Orphans of India", which was broadcast on NDTV Profit's Money Mantra on 8th August 2012.

He has been a guest speaker at various conferences like Franchise India Expo – the largest retail and franchise expo in India, Main Street Matters: Art of the Smart Start – a radio show on blogtalkradio, and has been featured on Deccan Chronicle.

He, presently, is busy with his marketing services company that helps brands with experiential marketing campaigns. When not working, he likes to watch cricket and indulge in various sports and physical activities. You can connect with him on http://vinilramdev.com or follow him on twitter at twitter.com/vinilramdev

# 15

## PUTTING 'SUE' IN SUCCESS

### - BY SUZANNA THERESIA, INTERNET MARKETER AND DIRECTOR AT EPHRAIM METTABEL.

**It Begins with the Creator.**

There will be no easy way to put it as always due to relentless judgment people stamp on people who believe in God, but I do believe in God and His might. And I'm not ashamed to put it so eloquently in the first few sentences of my part in this book since it's the foundation of how I even made it today.

Now that I've said that out the real life has waited me. God takes the first place in my life but that didn't work the magic for me, it's not witchcraft. Faith after all, is nothing without an action, and that is something that keeps me rolling.

Action; I was always a believer that action is all you need to get going. Taking the first step would be the determinant of where and how you are going next. Doing something is a lot better because you put your ideas and mind into something. You don't just dream about things and mind-plan everything and then just going back and forth on how you want to begin, you just do it. It allows you to be ahead of yourself and leaving you wanting to do more. So, action it is, the mantra, the mover, the measurement of the belief you invest within you, the commencement. A prove of a powerful existence in you, that allows you to act, one that you do have a control over but can't really work without a belief system that acts as the foundation. Without this power, we can't be sure on the direction we're going from the first action. Therefore, it is all possible only by God and His work of hand.

I have had my ups and downs too with taking action based on my belief system and faith, and to answer the title of this book, so my story begins.

**Being Perfect Takes Time.**

I would consider myself as a perfectionist. In my opinion, perfectionist would be a person who is far from the definition of perfect but then always looking for one. For me, I'd always set myself to be at the position that strives for perfection.

Taking action to me has always been a challenge on its own due to my perfectionist nature. I do believe that some other great minds in other pages of this book also had struggled the same thing too. In the past, I might have spent too many times in doing certain things, trying to get them perfect. But I have learned that in order to even getting close to perfection, an imperfect step must be taken.

This first step soon will develop into other steps, inch by inch taking you to the exact thing that motivates you to even take the first step. I myself was a living witness to the significance of first step, no matter how imperfect it was. You just got to walk a foot next to the other.

After wrapping up around the fact that we have move forward from where we were, to get things done is another part of the story. My perfectionism kicks in hard here at this part and it is both fun and frightening.

The fun part was that I went through so much brainstorming process and grew with it. I set a pretty high bar for myself and my judgment on

166

everything I work on. Not a single thing will be released for other's viewing if it doesn't pass the value control that based on my mind.

The not-so-fun part was how my time is wasted on just one task because I can't settle for anything less than nearing perfect. In my area, that means I will have to go over some products several times, bits by bits, just to shake the feeling that it is not enough. That causes me energy and gives enough stress. There's nothing effortless with being a perfectionist.

The time and energy I spent on a single thing also causes me my confidence. I can't be fearless and always tiptoe around my own thinking and my own action. Although simple for most people, this often scares me away from actually get things done. Indeed, it takes courage to show what we've got to people.

Everything I put into my work also causes me my leisure time. Even though I am not a workaholic and not planning to be any, it is simply unavoidable. This business and my forte can sometimes collide and time is not the biggest fan of this rendezvous.

I use to work for 15 to 18 hours a day. Now from the workaholic standpoint, I am definitely a strong candidate. But in my defense, I call that hardworking. I don't stop at the first sign of satisfaction, I choose to go over things several times because I realize that I'm in the business of making people assisted at all times and has a continuing maintenance afterwards. That doubles the amount of work I need, twice more than the work for a dead end product.

Because I don't believe easily, even if it is myself we are talking about, somehow people start to look at me as a reliable person. I mean, I do know that I am reliable, that's what I'm striving to be. Also, I'd always feel honored to have people invest their trust in me. But to receive such recognition that says: "Hey, I like you and what you do, so here's my time, resources, and energy, let's create something together", I'd call that something special. It takes courage to trust others, and if I have even the slightest chance to bear people who take risks to trust me, going back over a product a thousand times really seems like nothing.

Somewhere in between looking everything from the eyes of a perfectionist and being reliable at all times, the pressure is laid on. My life is a series of pressure. I'm pushing to the limit, every single time. I am hard at myself in a way that will make me humbled. Despite my lack of confidence, the pusher in me keeps going. It makes me understand that I will not achieve things easily, there's a process to it, a humbling one. After all, I am a firm believer of that old saying that says: "When you go easy on yourself, life will be hard on you. But, if you're hard on yourself, life will reward you with such an ease."

### The Need for Rock Bottom.

My name is Sue and I'm happy to say that I own several Internet Marketing products, three of them are Wordpress based, and continue to innovate to this day.

How do I get to the point when introducing myself brings such a content in my soul? Hitting rock bottom. I have explained how hard I can be on myself and how perfect I want everything to be, but I wasn't always like that. Before being where I'm now in my career, I was a settler. I nested and I used to pat my back in the morning convincing that what I was doing was enough for me. Turned out, it simply wasn't good enough.

I wasn't complaining or anything. I was even well aware that during my settling period, I did have a job of the dream. I lived in Singapore for the past 10 years, and approaching the year of 2009, something ate me up inside. I was really bored and unhappy with what I did, however beneficial it was. Sure it paid well, it leveraged the employee, and it had a big name and prestigious position for me, especially as a woman from the neighbor country. But I woke up and got up to work with no joy, feeling bombarded by office politics.

It soaks up happiness from my fibers, I felt like a 9 to 5 zombie, stuck within an unhealthy culture. This zombie couldn't even have a proper family vacation. Even for the local public holiday, the working clock is never stopped. Don't make me start on festive holidays. Going back to my hometown Indonesia was like visiting for the weekend, always only about 3 to 4 days. Sometimes I had to skip Christmas or New Year, I could only choose one and be okay with that. Well, I was not. I was at the bottom, holding everything together with the effort that I didn't enjoy.

It took me two years to weigh out all the options I had at the bottom. I could go on living a not gratifying career but still preserve my position and my income, with seeing family as the last thing on my mind, or I could put an end to everything and start over from scratch. If only I was looking for security, I might not be here today and I'd still be ping ponged as corporate slave by the political games within corporation. So, as I was built to do, I took action.

## Internet Marketing Realm.

2009 was a remark. I decided to explore my entrepreneurship side and got involved in Internet Marketing world. It has been a long time dream for me to finally be able to set my own business and doesn't work someone else's dream.

Hunch met guts, and the idea of controlling my time and space of work gave me the power to walk out of the company for good. I realized I can't learn and build something out of nothing with the person I was in the company. No time left for me to even think clearly if I had stayed there.

First time will always be the hardest, and that was the case as well. I didn't get the support I wanted and needed at that time, because in reality, a good, secure job is always the right option but just not for me. No real money can come from online business, that's what they told me. The 'no' was somewhat more overwhelming than the 'go ahead, do your thing', but that was something I'm truly thankful for today. Without those negativities, I may not have the motivation to make it successful.

Challenge fed me and the thought of actually creating something useful pushed me forward. Plus, people needed to tell you that you can't do it, or it won't work out like that, to make you embrace the idea that this is what you're supposed to be doing. I had that and it wasn't pretty, but hey, at least that sets me apart with the tenacious character and relentless willingness. That's what believers do, defying the stream.

As the choice of Internet Marketing, it was always been a personal interest. There was like a magnet that drawn me to it. What a great platform it was for me at that time, to start the ideas that I had. Online businesses were huge back in those days and still are to date, and there was a vision of future for me. When I learned about Internet Marketing, I thought this is a great platform for all the ideas I have. I can see the future of working and having an online business.

The problem was, I was a green rookie, with eyes wide open and an entrepreneurial knowledge of a freshman. I didn't know what I was supposed to do to build something online and call it my own. All I know that this was my solution to my freedom that I had a hunch that I was supposed to do this, no matter what.

I started all from zero. Now that I had my hunch supported me, my guts catapulted me back from the start. I did what I needed to do. I purchased any course I could get my hands on about Internet Marketing. It was pretty much a self-taught process that began to spinning out of control and making me overwhelmed. I couldn't pick out and eliminate things that I needed to learn and master. They came to me like they were one tornado after another.

Here's where we need more than just a hunch to survive. We need a clear vision. At that time, that was my safety net, my vision. No matter how reliable of a person I was, I needed someone else that would share my vision. I began to collect people and spend thousands of money on building software. I wasn't a programmer, that wasn't my area at all and I needed people to translate my idea into something tangible. Like the software itself, finding the right people was also a matter of trials and error with lots of money flying off of your account in the middle of the process.

I have had my share by being a victim of dishonest and irresponsible people and have learned my lesson. When bugs came out on the software, I have had people left me confused with no traces to be found. Thus, we need to find a commitment in the person we want to share a vision with. Above all, intelligence with no commitment is just a plain foolishness.

Negative people and quitters surrounded me the first year I tried to give birth to my product. The energy they brought at that time also drained me and left me with a profound loneliness. It was hard to keep on learning with the right determination and having people who didn't believe in you and walked out on you. I was asking myself: "What went wrong?" while trying not to entertain the idea of regret. I won't be regretful of life I had chosen.

As regret was off the table, I also never thought of giving up. That's just not how I would end it, not without a fight. I tried to find the silver linings in my loss. I thought to myself that I have learned things that would be profitable for me in the future. I might not see it yet, but I was alive and well, with new knowledge as my ammo. That alone would do it. That alone could get me back on my feet and shook off the lonely feeling.

**Products to Help.**

At last, the heart that endured shall see the fulfillment. I have come to know Wordpress, HTML, cpanel, and the online marketing design world as well as its structure, and now I have my own plugins. To get to this point required me a series of sacrifices, from money, time, and good night sleeps. I thank God that I may say that I persisted and refused to back down.

From a timid beginning by affiliating with ClickBank, learning about Free Traffic until actually owning traffic exchange sites called Rainbow-Traffic.com and Shinelight-Traffic.com with more unique take than the competitors, I had evolved to become a product creator. My first successful product was Smart Graphic Designer or smartdesignit. The product was made to help internet marketers using graphic software with easier approach.

From that point on, the hard work paid off. Exactly two years ago, InstaBuilder, the Wordpress plugins that I created was launched and I can't ask for anything better. I was able to also develop InstaMember and InstaTheme. They were then quickly followed by a PLR membership that helps the marketers to copyright their plugins called InstaProduct. Starting off with nothing, I can say now that I am a product of my action, my first step, and I make a living out of my passion.

The key word in all products that I was lucky to develop is "help". My goal all along was to create something that will help people becoming more innovative, a site where people can go and start something on their own, a site that is easy to use, easy to be learned, and intuitive. People can reap benefits out of my products with sensible price.

All of the Insta platforms are there to make all fellow internet marketers enjoy what they are doing and become successful at it. I am familiar with the struggle, and for people who are new, my products can give them ease price and product wise. It is never easy to have something successful on your own and in online space, and to know that I help them even in the simplest form, is enough.

I must say that being able to do what you love and knowing that people respond to what you do positively is both humbling and rewarding. When I know a customer feels helped by the existence of any of my products, I am able to say that all the failure and delayed success were worth it. People whom I knew along the journey, whether it's the people whom I worked with or the people I learned from, even the people who bought my products were all contributing and shaping who Sue is right now.

### Never Looking Back.

Success for me is prosperity in all things and be in good health as it is stated so truthfully in John 3:2. Success is having your life under control with you as the controller, and not the circumstances around you. Success is achieving something that you have planned to do, from making a business idea a reality to simply spending time with your family whenever you plan to. That is what I called success.

I am a hero for my surrounding, and this kind of success motors me and keeps me sane. I do think I am successful now that I have full control of my life and my time. This condition allows me to share with others all things I might not be able to do if I were to stay in the corporate doing things that I don't love. I am blessed, my family is blessed, and I think it can be classified as heroic since I can alter the lives I need to change.

A dreamer is wide-awake and focused, always looking for the next move. A dreamer is someone who's not afraid to learn all over again just for the sake of knowledge. If you too, are a dreamer and have been carrying something inside of you that you believe in, take that first step of faith. Take that measure and walk the path by keeping yourself inspired by others who have done it. Put your stamp in the things you want to do and don't let the negativity overpowers you!

My websites:

http://www.SuzannaTheresia.com
http://www.smartdesignit.com
http://instabuilder.com
http://instamember.com
http://instatheme.com
http://insta-product.com

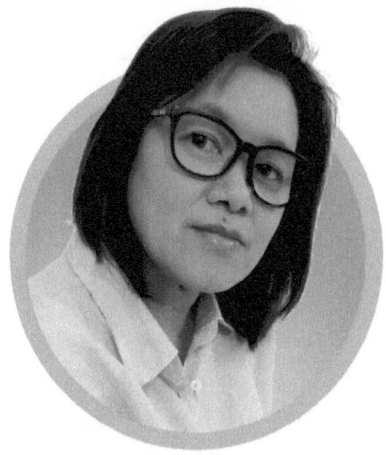

## Suzanna Theresia

I am Suzanna Theresia and my friends call me Sue. I am originally from Indonesia but landed in Singapore where I have lived for the past 10 years.

I'm an Internet Marketer and Product Creator. I began my journey in Internet marketing in 2009, and have been doing it full time since 2011.

I started as an affiliate to some Clickbank products. From one eBook I learned about Free Traffic, and I got to know about Traffic Exchanges Industry. I then owned 2 traffic exchange sites; Rainbow-Traffic.com and Shinelight-Traffic.com. I bought a script and customized it – I make my 2 TE sites unique – we added unique features, unique designs etc.

Things were going well, and I had a little success with the traffic exchanges. But I've always felt that there is something else I could do better, so after 2 years I moved to product creation.

My first product is Smart Graphic Designer –http://smartdesignit.com, it's an easy-to use graphic software designed for internet marketers.

I now own 2 Wordpress plugins and 1 Wordpress theme; namely InstaBuilder, InstaMember. And InstaTheme. I also own a PLR membership where we deliver a brand new plugin complete with PLR rights each month; namely InstaProduct. I focus on product creation and list building. My passion is developing products and sites that are innovative, easy to use, easy to learn, and intuitive. I have found my passion and never looked back.

# 16

## GONE NATIVE!

- BY KEITH KIRWEN, FOUNDER AND TRAVEL BLOGGER AT
KEITHKIRWEN.COM

Being one of the few native English speakers in the area often has its benefits. This weekend was one of those cases. I had been hired to be the master of ceremonies and translator for the European Mountain Meeting in my adopted home of the Val d'Aran.

We had been preparing for this great event full of conferences by world-renowned mountaineers and adventurers and the day had finally arrived. There were people flying in from all over; from the United States, Russia, Italy, Australia, England and of course a lot of people were coming from Spain. I was psyched. I love the rush of being on stage and the show was just about to begin.

As I was setting up the microphone, the director of the event, Gabriela, hurried up to me saying, "Keith, Leo has just arrived from the UK and needs to get something to eat before his conference. Please take him somewhere for dinner and hurry back. We'll take care of setting up the stage." Leo was scheduled to be the main speaker of the night and I had to translate for him! As I headed off, Gabriela shouted, "Leo is the good looking blonde haired guy out front."

Finding Leo was easy. You can tell an extreme sportsman when you see one. We met and quickly headed off to one of Vielha's best tapas bars, Urtau, for a quick and tasty dinner. I knew very little about him and since I was going to be sharing the stage with him translating his story and adventures this was the perfect moment to learn more. His life was full of amazing extreme adventures climbing big mountains, big wall rock climbing and all kinds of crazy base-jumping. He told me that he would be presenting his most recent movie this evening in the conference. I was impressed.

As most people do when they meet me here in Spain he soon asked, "Keith, what are you doing here?" "How did you end up in this little mountain valley in the middle of the Pyrenees?" I looked at my watch to make sure we had enough time. I had told my personal adventure story before and knew it took a while.

"It's kind of a long story really, but since you've asked and we have some time I'll tell you how a boy who grew up in Tennessee ended up living in the world's greatest place. First, I have to give you a bit of background.

"It all really started when I was a young kid camping and water skiing with my family on the weekends and in the summers. I have such fond memories of setting up camp, gathering firewood, starting and watching over the fires, hiking in the forest with my family during the days and even at night with homemade torches and water skiing all day. I always felt something special about being in nature.

Somehow, even as a young boy I knew that I "felt better" or was more at peace when I was outdoors. This was also magnified during my years in the Boy Scouts. Year after year I would learn about nature and every summer we would go on campouts and hikes. It was in the Scouts that I first went backpacking and experienced the joy of being able to camp and hike and move in the mountains without any contact with city things like cars and machines and noise. It was then that somehow the mountain presented itself to me as a place of peace. A therapeutic place, if you will."

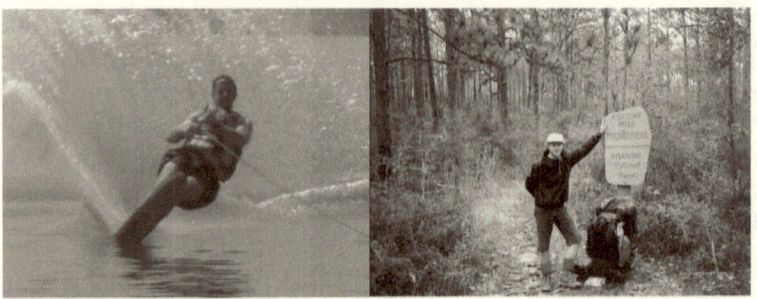

"So, I lived a pretty normal suburban life in the United States. I went to private Catholic schools and played all kinds of sports and after I graduated from high school I went off to university and decided to study marketing.

I really didn't know what I wanted to do. My first year or so at school was a real fiasco; too much partying and too little studying. So I went back to my hometown and enrolled in the University of Memphis.

I decided to do a series of aptitude tests to see if I could get some inspiration for my future studies and professional career. The results that came back suggested that a good career match for me would be that of a Social Worker. I did some investigation and learned that I could study to become a counselor or psychotherapist and later combine my love for the outdoors working in wilderness environments helping people transform and improve their lives.

I liked that idea and quickly enrolled in the program. I graduated and immediately began working in the outdoors with troubled youth in Tennessee.

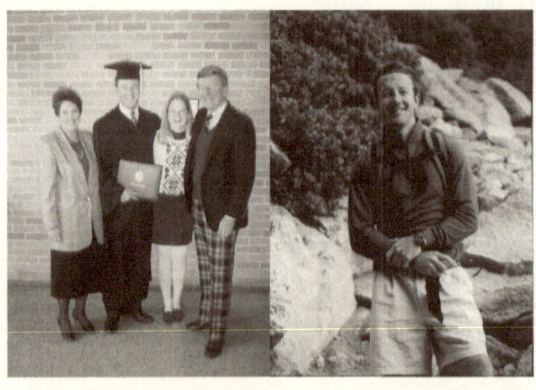

A couple years later I got a job in Montana working as a wilderness guide and therapist in a center for young men with problems with addictions. You may not know it, but America is quite big. It took my father and I, and my dog, 48 hours non-stop driving to get from Memphis to Montana.

"Are you still with me?"

"Yes, please continue. This sounds like it is going to get interesting."

"Having grown up in the south I never had seen much snow and had never been on a big mountain. In Montana I learned to snowboard. Learning to snowboard was a real thrill for me and in fact it changed my life, forever.

I am here with you today because of the snowboard. I became obsessed with the sport. All I could do was think about boarding all throughout the year. I remember hiking down mountain paths in the summer imagining they were full of snow and I would pretend I was riding down the mountain jumping this and jumping that or turning here or turning there.

My job as a wilderness guide and therapist was really amazing. I spent hundreds of days in the backcountry helping young men turn their lives around. It was really fantastic because we would climb mountains, build snow caves, weather -20° to -40° winters, fish for trout in high mountain lakes in the summer, and hike 6 to 8 hours a day all the while doing therapy. The mountain is really powerful, as I am sure you know. I read your bio sheet and know you have a lot of experience in the mountains."

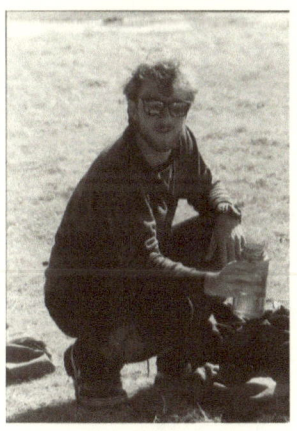

"Could you tell me about one of your experiences working with the kids?"

"Of course, on one winter expedition we got lost in the wilderness. My co-worker and I had misread the map and when we realized where we were it was too late for us to climb the mountain peak we had intended to climb on that trip.

The trips were pretty intense. We would spend around 16 days on top of the snow without tents, without fires and using short skis to pull our sleds across the rolling mountain terrain. Well, on this occasion we needed to come up with a plan to create a 'peak experience' for our clients.

We decided to set up camp and for one full day the 10 of us piled snow with our snow shovels until we had made huge mound of snow. It was probably 5 meters long (16 feet), 3 meters wide (10 feet) and 3 meters tall.

We waited until the next day to allow the snow to settle and then dug out the snow from the inside. By this time of the trip we were a well-organized team and we worked together to hollow out the mountain of snow thereby creating our own snow cave. We spent the next two nights sleeping in there together. It was really amazing. The kids were ecstatic about setting up camp inside a snow cave that they had made!

There are many more stories of personal transformation I could tell you about, but it would take too much time right now. I'll be happy to share them with you another moment."

"Do you want me to continue telling you about me coming to Spain?"

"Please!"

"So, at this point I was very happy with my life. I was spending all my time in the mountains both in my free time and at work. I was snowboarding, rock climbing, trail running, mountain biking and trekking. It was fantastic, but it wasn't enough. I wanted to do something more exciting. Something more 'earth shaking' if you will. It was then that I decided to make a big change in my life and follow the slogan of Nike. You know, "Just Do It!""

"What did you do mate? That sounds pretty serious."

"In a nutshell, Leo, I quit my job, sold everything I owned except my mountaineering and snowboarding gear and bought a 1972 VW bus with the plan of living in it with my dog, Teva, at the base of the Whistler/Blackcomb ski resort in Canada. I had saved about ten grand and wanted to spend one winter snowboarding every day, not just on my days off. I was 25 years old."

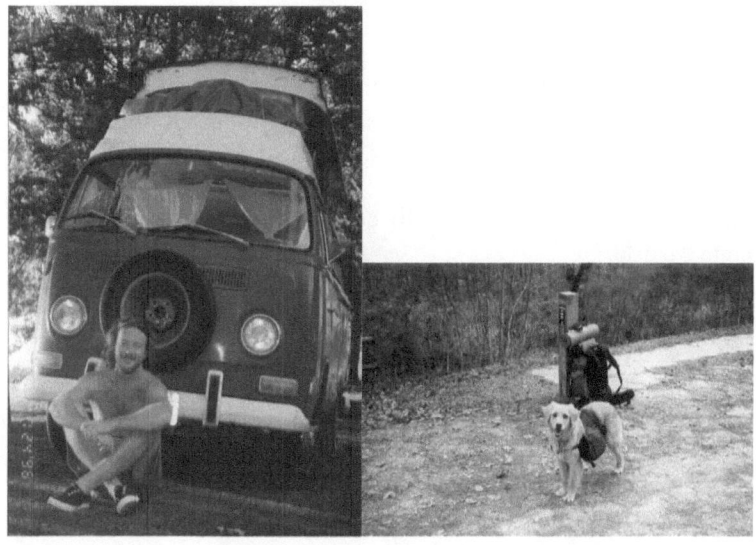

"Wow, then what happened? How did you get here from there?"

"Let me take you back to the moment where this whole life/snowboard adventure really took off. Imagine, if you will, that you are with me at my house in Montana back in 1995. I am in my garage with Teva packing my gear."

"I have recently taken my bus and parked it on cement blocks at my girlfriend's grandfather's farm. Everything I own that I can't carry with me is inside the bus. My plans have changed. I'm not going to Canada in my bus, but rather to Spain by plane. I turn to Teva as she lowers her head and sits down next to me and say to her, 'Don't worry girl, Genio is going to take good care of you. I know you're sad because I'm packing my bags again'.

At that moment my housemate and co-worker, Genio, walks in and says, 'Are you sure you know what you're doing man. I mean I understood when you sold everything you owned, quit your job and bought the bus, but this is a bit extreme! You're going to Spain? You don't even speak Spanish and you hardly know anyone there!'

'You're right, I don't, but I couldn't be happier than I am right now', "I responded with a big smile on my face and joy running through my veins."

'You don't know where you're going to stay or anything. How long are you gonna be gone?', "he questioned."

"I looked at him, looked at Teva, looked at my gear and after a moment's pause, (I had yet to really think about this) I responded, 'I don't know how long I'll be gone.' "I looked into his eyes and said", 'Perhaps a week, a month, the winter or maybe the rest of my life.'

"The next day I said goodbye to both of them and a few days later I landed in Madrid."

"Mate, that is phenomenal. Why did you decide to do all that? Why did you decide to come to Spain of all places to snowboard?"

"You know at that moment in my life I wanted something else. I wanted more adventure. My life was full of adventure, but it wasn't profound enough. I wanted to shake the roots of my being and discover what life would be like trusting completing in the universe. I wanted to let go of everything I knew which was keeping me grounded. I wanted a personal and revolutionary transformation.

Life was great. I wasn't running from anything, but rather towards something and the snowboard was the excuse. I came to Spain because I had met a couple from Spain on a trip in West Africa, after I had quit my job, and I learned from them that there were plenty of options for snowboarding in Spain."

"So, you have essentially, Gone Native, haven't you?

"I guess you could say that I have Gone Native, but never really thought about it that way."

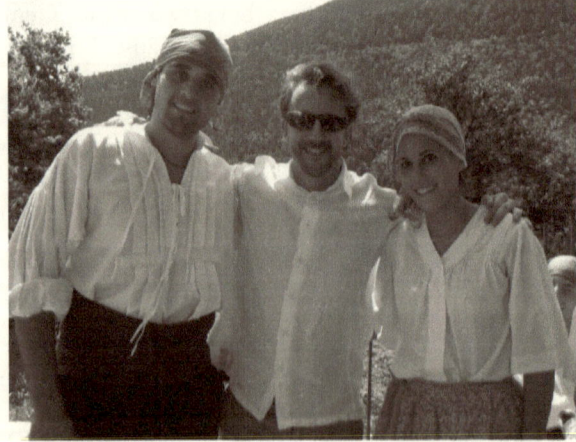

"How did you get from Madrid to this little hidden place called the Val d'Aran?"

"We don't really have enough time now Leo for me to tell more about me. I don't want to bore you anyway".

"Bore me! Hell, you've got me on the edge of my seat. I want to hear the rest of the story. It sounds like a movie."

"We've gotta go. Let me go pay and we'll head back to the conference. On the way back I want to tell you about this amazing Aran Valley. This weekend, if you really want, I'll tell you the rest of my arrival story".

"Dinner's paid - vamanos. So, as I was saying, I want to tell you about this place. I don't know if you realize it, but you've come to Southern Europe's top mountain destination, the Val d'Aran. We are in the northwest corner of the autonomous region of Spain known as Catalonia. Barcelona is the capital and is about 4 hours from here on the Mediterranean coast. This hidden treasure of a mountain valley is truly unique for a number of reasons; one being that the people here have their own language, culture and history."

"They have their own language?"

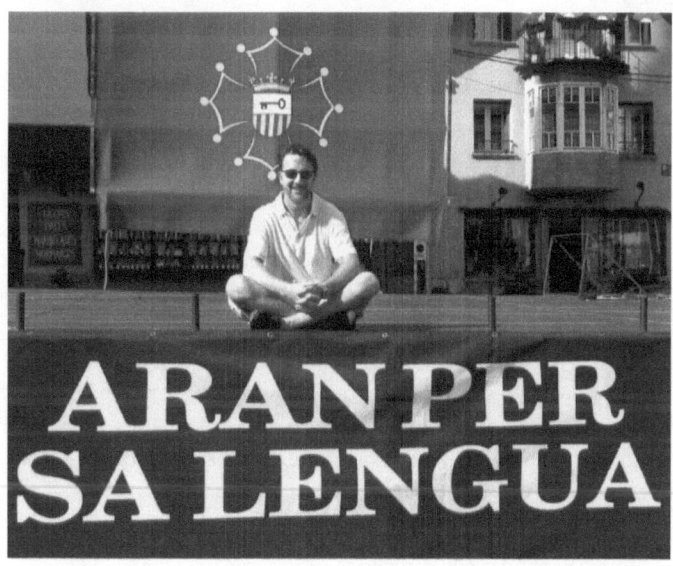

"Yes, it's called Aranese and it comes from the Middle Ages. I've come to know and love the people here. Most of them speak four languages:

Aranese, Catalan, Spanish and English or French. Pretty amazing really considering that you and I come from largely monolingual countries. Well anyway, as I was telling you, this valley is really awesome.

The economy here is based largely on tourism. We've got the best ski resort of Southern Europe, Baqueira Beret, as our flagship enterprise. But, there is so much more than downhill skiing and snowboarding here. You name it for winter sports - we've got it. Have you ever been heli-skiing?"

"No I haven't, but have always dreamed of doing it!"

"Well, we're home to a World class heli-skiing operation also. There's dog sledding, snowshoeing, snowmobiling, cross country skiing and ski mountaineering…the list goes on and on."

"Outside of the winter season this is a trail running, mountain biking and hiking paradise. I know you love sports. There are literally hundreds of kilometers of mountain trails.

The food here is really spectacular also. We have one of the world's best collections of Romanesque architecture. I can't get enough of this place and I love sharing it with the world. Because the Val d'Aran is largely unknown on the global travel scene it is still wonderfully authentic and not over run with tourists.

After this weekend, you'll have to let me help you organize a trip here with your wife. You'll love it too."

"Sounds amazing! I'll definitely have to come back. Now you've left me hanging Keith. Tomorrow you've gotta finish your story. Okay?"

"Okay, okay! No problem, tomorrow we're scheduled to go on a hike with the participants of the conference. I'll be translating for you. We'll have time, for me to tell you the rest."

"Okay great. Now it's time to focus on the conference. Are you ready to translate for me? Don't worry about the camera flashes! You'll get used to it. It's gonna be fun. The movie is really fast paced and full of action. Here's your microphone."

"You bet I'm ready! Let's do it!"

"Ladies and Gentlemen. Señoras y Señores. Welcome to the European

Mountain Meeting. It is our pleasure to introduce to you our opening night speaker, the one and only, Leo Houlding, straight from the United Kingdom. Welcome Leo! The stage is all yours."

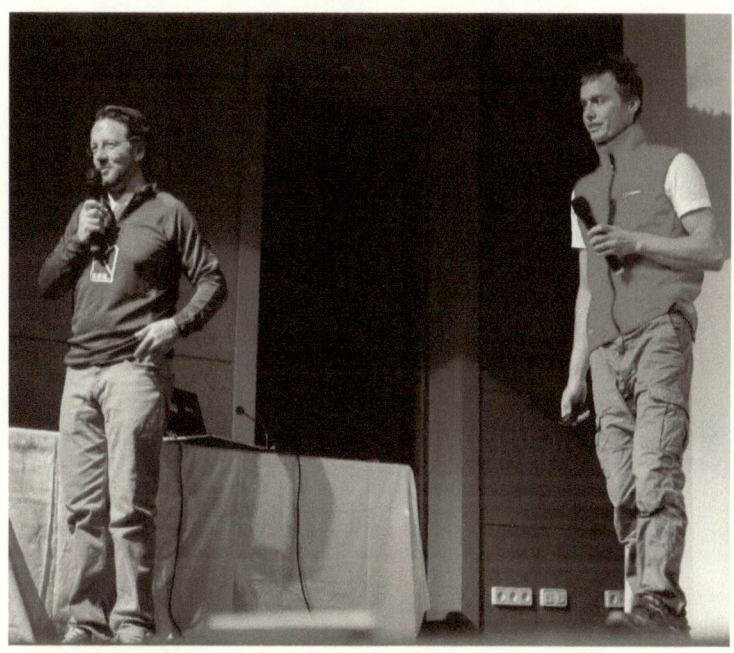

*Thank you kindly for taking the time to read a bit about me and my story. This chapter is just a glimpse into my life and the lessons and stories I have to share. I would be happy to have you download a free chapter from my book, The World's Greatest Place, where you can read about all the amazing events that took place to bring me to the Val d'Aran and Catalonia. When you download the free chapter, you will be put on a list to be notified when I publish this book and my up-and-coming book, The Mountain is My Therapist.

You may also wish to download any of my free e-books on the same web page. Please click here for the downloads:
http://www.keithkirwen.com/ebooks/

Learn more about Keith and his travel destination:

Web Page:
http://www.keithkirwen.com

Social Media:

http://www.youtube.com/keithkirwentv

http://www.facebook.com/keithkirwenn

https://www.linkedin.com/in/keithkirwen

http://www.twitter.com/keithkirwen

http://www.googleplus.com/keithkirwen

http://www.instagram.com/keithkirwen

http://www.pinterest.com/keithkirwen

30-minute interview about "Inbound Destination Travel Blogging" by Keith Kirwen

http://www.keithkirwen.com/thought-leaders-chat-video-interview/

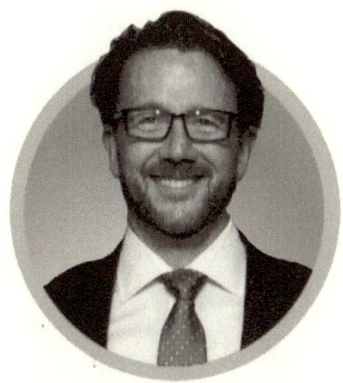

Keith Kirwen is a Chicago born man-of-many-hats who at young ripe age of 25, three years after graduating from the University of Memphis, Tennessee, quit his career as a therapist and wilderness guide in northwest Montana selling everything he owned except his dog and his mountaineering and snowboarding gear.

He bought an old hippy Volkswagen bus to spend a winter snowboarding in Canada. His spirit of adventure took him, instead, to find love, passion, business and adventure in a foreign land. He never returned.

He is a serial enthusiast inspiring others to reach their highest potential. From owner of a successful language school in the Pyrenees Mountains, to a short career as a Yoga instructor Keith has recently written his first published book, The World's Greatest Place, which is the story of personal transformation and discovery in a foreign land.

He will soon publish his second book, The Mountain is My Therapist, from which he has created a motivational, sensorial and interactive conference. Speaker and translator, Keith is now a travel destination video blogger dedicating his time to sharing his beloved and adopted home, Catalonia, to the world.

When Keith isn't working on his next project he enjoys traveling the world with his spouse, trail running with his dogs and skiing and snowboarding.

Much of his work can be appreciated visiting his web and social media platforms at www.keithkirwen.com

# ABOUT THE AUTHORS

This is a book written by industry experts, each contributing a chapter. Here's a list of all the CO-AUTHORS of this publication (in no particular order):

Xesco Espar
David Spungin
Jashvant Shah
Dr. Joanne Messenger
Abe Cherian
Greg Hague
Stephanie Mulac
Axel Meierhoefer

Frankie Mooney
Daniel Van Neikerk
Ellie Borden
Shelly-Ann Williams
Dr. Debbie Novick
Vinil Ramdev
Suzanna Theresia
Keith Kirwen

Published by: Raam Anand